Michael M. Dediu

Hippocrates to Fleming:
Medicine History
celebrated after 1943

A chronological and photographic documentary

DERC Publishing House
Tewksbury (Boston), Massachusetts, U. S. A.

Copyright ©2019 by Michael M. Dediu

Published and printed in the
United States of America
On the Great Seal of the United States are included:
E Pluribus Unum (Out of many, one)
Annuit Coeptis (He has approved of the undertakings)
Novus Ordo Seclorum (New order of the ages)

Library of Congress Control Number: 2019901584

Dediu, Michael M.

Hippocrates to Fleming: Medicine History celebrated after 1943
A chronological and photographic documentary

ISBN-13: 978-1-939757-85-2

Preface

The physicians and the medicine in general play an essential role our civilization, and it is a great pleasure to remember and celebrate them, looking from a recent perspective.

I dedicate this succinct medicine history, with much gratitude, to the very dedicated physicians who help me over the years – I will mention here, in alphabetical order, those who I remember (I apologize for not remembering those who helped me in my childhood, and others who helped me occasionally): Dr. Peter Barley, Dr. Bita, Dr. Dimescu, Dr. Milton Drake, Dr. Dumitrescu, Dr. Jason Efstathiou, D. Phil., Dr. Adam Feldman, Dr. Allan Goldstein, Dr. Scott Greenstein, Prof. Dr. Paul Huang, Dr. Richard Johnson, Dr. Veikko Koivisto, Ph. D., Dr. John Loewenstein, Dr. Scott McDougal, Dr. Alec Meleger, Dr. George Palade, Ph. D., Nobel Prize, Dr. Popescu, Dr. Pupo, Prof. Dr. Harry Rubash, Dr. Paul Shellito, Dr. Leonard Tom.

Starting from 1943, in a chronological order, we present the medicine history, which was commemorated in the last 75 years. There are also many attractive and historic photographs – I want to thank my wife for her assistance.

This book, for the general public, reminds us of the famous quote of Voltaire about medical doctors and their assistants: **"People who are occupied in the restoration of health to other people, by the joint exertion of skill and humanity, are above all the great of the Earth. They even partake of divinity, since to preserve and renew is almost as noble as to create."**

Michael M. Dediu, Ph. D.

Tewksbury (Boston), U. S. A., 28 February 2019

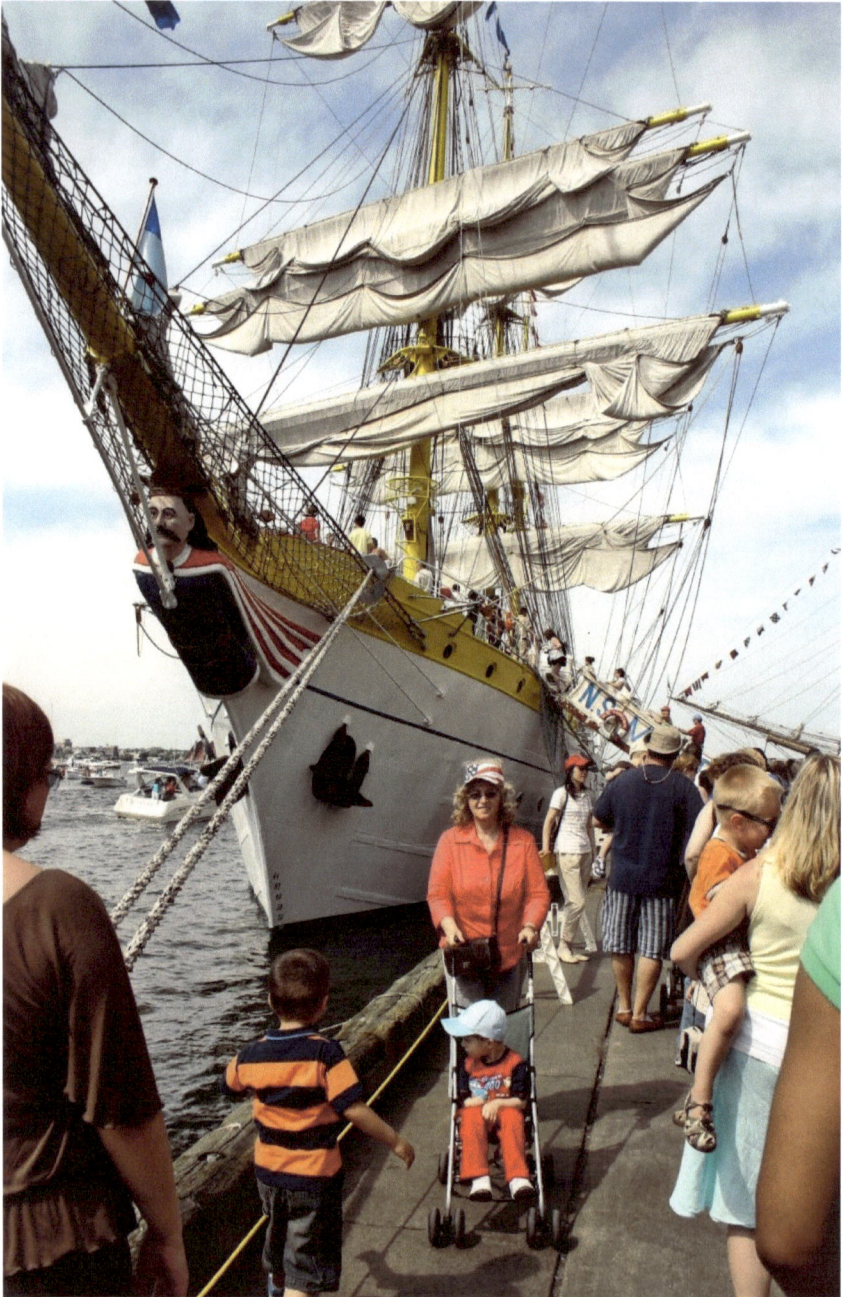

11 July 2009, tall ship at the northwest side of Boston Fish Pier in Boston (1630, population 650,000) Harbor (Port of Boston has 200 ha, draft depth 12 m, 237,000 containers/year; the Boston Harborwalk provides public access to much of the harbor's edge).

Table of Contents

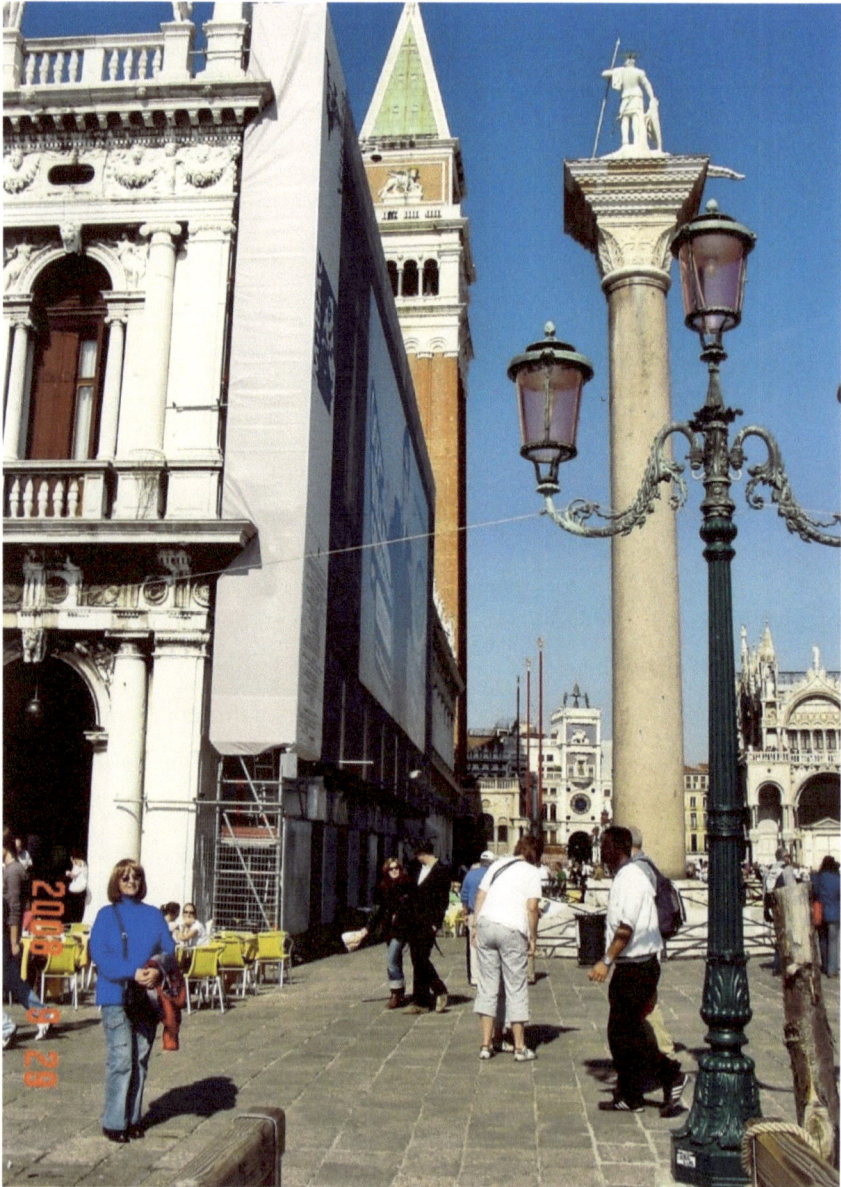

29 September 2008, Venezia (421), Piazza San Marco (1084) Libreria Sansoviniana. (1468-1560, left), Campanile (850, 1514, 1912, 99 m, back), Torre dell'Orologio (1499, back), San Theodore Column (1268), Basilica di San Marco (1156-1173, right).

Chapter 1. 1943 – 1952: Diocles of Carystus, Sylvius, Jenner, Koch, Fleming

1943 – Golgi, Hunt, Roberts, Dam, Doisy

- 400 years ago, in 1543, **Jacobus Sylvius** observed the centripetal movement of the venous bloodstream, from the structure and arrangement of valves in the veins. Before it had been believed that blood flowed outwards to the periphery, even in the veins.

- 4 January – 300th anniversary of the birth of Sir **Isaac Newton** (4 Jan 1643 – 31 March 1727, aged 84.2), great English mathematician, astronomer, theologian, author and physicist.

- 14 January - **Ralph M. Steinman** was born (14 January 1943, Montreal, Canada – 30 Sep 2011, of cancer, aged 68.6), Canadian-born American Professor at Rockefeller University, New York, NY, USA. He received the Nobel Prize in Physiology or Medicine in 2011, 3 days after his death, "for his discovery, in 1973 (age 30), of the dendritic cell and its role in adaptive immunity".

- 19 February - **Tim Hunt** was born (19 February 1943, Neston, United Kingdom), British Researcher at Imperial Cancer Research Fund, London, United Kingdom. He received the Nobel Prize in Physiology or Medicine in 2001, at the age of 58, together with Leland Hartwell and Sir Paul Nurse.

- 26 June - **Karl Landsteiner**, Foreign Member of the Royal Society, Austrian-born biologist, physician, and immunologist, passed away at the age of 75 years and 12 days (14 June 1868, Baden bei Wien, Austrian Empire – 26 June 1943, The Rockefeller University, New York City, NY, USA). He distinguished the main blood groups in 1900, at age 32, having developed the modern system of classification of blood groups. In 1901 Karl Landsteiner,

33, introduces the system to classify blood into A, B, AB, and O groups. In 1930, Landsteiner, 62, was awarded the Nobel Prize for his description of the human ABO blood group system.

7 July – 100 years ago, in 1843, **Camillo Golgi** was born (7 July 1843, Corteno, Italy - 21 January 1926, Pavia, Italy, aged 82.5), Italian Professor at Pavia University, Pavia, Italy. He received the Nobel Prize in Physiology or Medicine in 1906, with **Santiago Ramón y Cajal**, in recognition of their work on the structure of the nervous system - in the 1870s Camillo Golgi discovered that nerve cells could be stained with silver nitrate. This led to groundbreaking studies of how the nervous system is structured and functions.

- 6 September - **Richard J. Roberts** was born (6 September 1943, Derby, United Kingdom), British-born American Researcher at New England Biolabs, Beverly, MA, USA. He received the Nobel Prize in Physiology or Medicine in 1993, at the age of 50, together with Philip A. Sharp, "for their discoveries of split genes."

- 6 November – The author was born.

- 11 December - 100th anniversary of the birth of **Heinrich Hermann Robert Koch** (11 December 1843, Kingdom of Hanover – 27 May 1910, Baden-Baden, Germany, aged 66.4), German physician and microbiologist. As the founder of modern bacteriology, he identified the specific causative agents of tuberculosis, cholera, and anthrax, and gave experimental support for the concept of infectious disease. He received the Nobel Prize in Physiology or Medicine in 1905.

- **Selman A. Waksman**, 55, (22 July 1888, Nova Prylika, Kiev, Russia – 16 August 1973, Woods Hole, Falmouth, MA, USA, aged 85), Russian-born, American inventor, biochemist and microbiologist, discovered in 1943, at Rutgers University, the antibiotic streptomycin, for which he received the Nobel Prize in Physiology or Medicine in 1952, at age 64.

- The Nobel Prize in Physiology or Medicine 1943 was awarded to **Henrik Carl Peter Dam**, 48 (21 February 1895,

Copenhagen, Denmark - 17 April 1976, Copenhagen, Denmark, aged 81.1), Danish Professor at Polytechnic Institute, Copenhagen, Denmark, for his discovery of vitamin K in 1934 (that is needed for the blood to coagulate; this knowledge became especially important in treating bleeding among small children), and **Edward Adelbert Doisy,** 50 (13 November 1893, Hume, IL, USA - 23 October 1986, St. Louis, MO, USA, aged 92 years 11 months and 10 days), American Professor at Saint Louis University, St. Louis, MO, USA, for his discovery of the chemical nature of vitamin K - in 1939 Edward Doisy produced two variants of vitamin K in pure form, allowing him to determine its structure and, to produce it by artificial means.

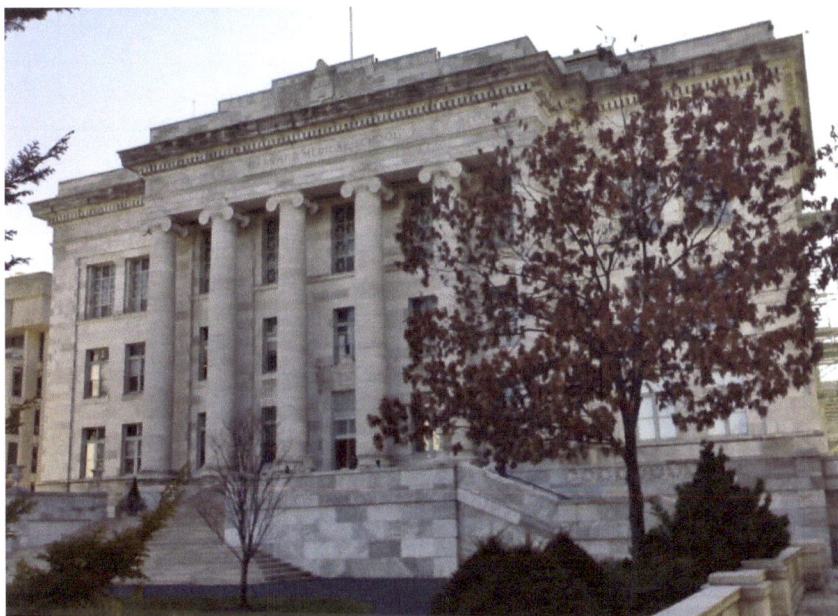

3 Dec 2009, the northeast façade of the Harvard Medical School Anno Domini 1904, founded in 1782, the graduate medical school of Harvard University, 1660 students, acceptance rate 3.7%.

1944 – Rynd, Avery, Erlanger, Gasser

- 100 years ago, in 1844, Irish physician **Francis Rynd**, 43, (1801 – 1861, aged 60) invented a hollow hypodermic needle to make the first recorded subcutaneous injections, specifically of a sedative to treat neuralgia.

- **Oswald Avery**, 67, (21 October 1877 – 20 February 1955, aged 77.3, Canadian-American physician and medical researcher) proved that DNA is the bearer of organisms' genetic code.

- The Nobel Prize in Physiology or Medicine 1944 was awarded to **Joseph Erlanger**, 70 (5 January 1874, San Francisco, CA, USA - 5 December 1965, St. Louis, MO, USA, aged 91 years and 11 months), American Professor at Washington University, St. Louis, MO, USA, and **Herbert Spencer Gasser**, 56 (5 July 1888, Platteville, WI, USA - 11 May 1963, New York, NY, USA, aged 74.9), American Professor at Rockefeller Institute for Medical Research, New York, NY, USA, for their discoveries relating to the highly differentiated functions of single nerve fibers - in 1922, in collaboration with Gasser, Erlanger adapted the cathode-ray oscillograph for the study of nerve action potentials.

1945 – Volta, Röntgen, Fleming, Chain, Florey

- 18 February - 200th anniversary of the birth of **Alessandro Volta** (18 Feb 1745, Como, Duchy of Milano – 5 March 1827, Como, Lombardia-Venezia, aged 82 years and 15 days), Italian inventor of the battery in 1799, when he was 54, and now, thanks to the work of scientists and engineers, the batteries are intensely used for medical applications, and continue to dramatically improve.

Lithium-ion batteries have become the most common rechargeable batteries for consumer electronics and automotive applications, due to their high energy densities, decent power density, relatively high cell voltages, and low weight-to-volume ratios. The increased demand, and the pressure for improving battery performance, have intensified the need for mathematical modeling. Modeling and simulations allow for the analysis of an almost unlimited number of design parameters and operating conditions, at a relatively small cost. Experimental tests are used to provide the necessary validation of the models.

The deep freeze in the U.S., in the week of 28 January 2019, exposed some of the limitations of electric vehicles. Owners of Tesla, Nissan and Jaguar EVs reported a loss of range of as much as 30%, amid the recording-setting low temperatures associated with the Polar Vortex. The problem is that lithium-ion batteries, in general, are most efficient at about 20° C. Still, there is optimism that the next generation of EV batteries will dramatically improve performance, although "solid state" batteries aren't expected to be mass produced until 2022 at the earliest.

27 March - 100th anniversary of the birth of **Wilhelm Conrad Röntgen** (27 March 1845, Lennep, Prussia (now Remscheid, Germany) – 10 Feb 1923, Munich, Germany, aged 77.9), German mechanical engineer and physicist, who, on 8 November 1895, at age 50.6, produced and detected electromagnetic radiation in a wavelength range known as X-rays or Röntgen rays, which became important in medical diagnosis and therapy, an achievement that earned him the first Nobel Prize in Physics in 1901, at age 56.

- The Nobel Prize in Physiology or Medicine 1945 was awarded to Sir **Alexander Fleming**, 64 (6 August 1881, Lochfield, Scotland - 11 March 1955, London, United Kingdom, aged 73.6, buried in St. Paul's Cathedral), British Professor at London University, London, United Kingdom, **Ernst Boris Chain**, 39 (19 June 1906, Berlin, Germany - 12 August 1979, Mulrany, Ireland, aged 73.1), German-born British Professor at University of Oxford, Oxford, United Kingdom, and Sir **Howard Walter Florey**, 47 (24 September 1898, Adelaide, Australia - 21 February 1968, Oxford, United Kingdom, aged 69.4), Australian-born British Professor at University of Oxford, Oxford, United Kingdom, for the discovery of penicillin by Sir Alexander Fleming in 1928, and Ernst Boris Chain and Howard Florey succeeded in systematically producing a pure form of penicillin, at the beginning of the 1940s, and in investigating its properties in more detail. Additional efforts led to a pharmaceutical that could be produced in larger quantities, with curative effect in various infectious diseases.

- The first vaccine for influenza was developed.

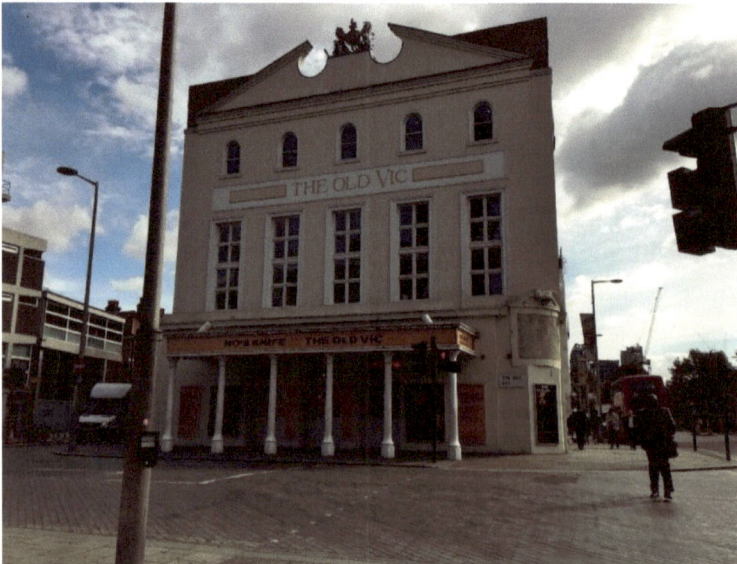

London: The northwest façade of the Old Vic Theatre (1818, 1871, 1902, 1927, 1938, 1950, 1960, 1963, 1985, 2003, 1067 capacity), on the corner of The Cut and Waterloo Rd., a traditional playhouse with big name actors (Laurence Olivier (1907-1989)) and top directors.

1946 – Hoffmann, Tatum, Muller

- 8 February - **Felix Hoffmann** passed away at the age of 78 years and 18 days (21 Jan 1868, Ludwigsburg, Germany – 8 Feb 1946, Switzerland). In 1897, at the age of 29, in a two-week period, while working at Bayer, the German chemist Felix Hoffmann synthesized both aspirin and diamorphine (heroin). Aspirin is one of the most widely beneficial drugs ever.

- **Fritz Lipmann**, 47, discovered the substance that, along with a protein, forms an enzyme that facilitates an important step in cell metabolism. He described its role, and gave it the name coenzyme A. He received the Nobel Prize in Physiology or Medicine in 1953.

- **Joshua Lederberg** and **Edward Tatum** demonstrated in 1946 that bacteria's genes can also change in a way similar to that of sexual reproduction seen in more complex organisms. Bacteria can go through a phase in which two bacteria exchange genetic material with one another by passing pieces of DNA across a bridge-like connection. Joshua Lederberg also proved the phenomenon known as transduction, in which DNA is transferred between bacteria via bacteriophages.

- The Nobel Prize in Physiology or Medicine 1946 was awarded to **Hermann Joseph Muller**, 56 (21 December 1890, New York, NY, USA - 5 April 1967, Indianapolis, IN, USA, aged 76.3), American Professor at Indiana University, Bloomington, IN, USA, for the discovery, in 1927, of the production of mutations by means of X-ray irradiation - the number of genetic mutations observed in fruit flies increased when they were exposed to x-rays. He found that the higher the dose of x-rays and other ionizing radiation the flies were exposed to, the greater the number of mutations that occurred.

1947 – Simpson, Wright, Cori

- 4 November – 100 years ago, in 1847, **James Young Simpson,** 37, (7 June 1811 – 6 May 1870, aged 58.9, Scottish obstetrician), discovered the anesthetic properties of chloroform, and first uses it, successfully, on a patient, in an obstetric case in Edinburgh.

- 30 April - Sir **Almroth Edward Wright,** British bacteriologist and immunologist passed away at the age of 85.6 (10 Aug 1861, Middleton Tyas, Yorkshire, England — 30 April 1947, Farnham Common, Buckinghamshire, England). In 1896, at age 35, developed a system of anti-typhoid fever inoculation, recognizing early on that antibiotics would create resistant bacteria, and being a strong advocate for preventive medicine.

- The Nobel Prize in Physiology or Medicine 1947 was awarded to Carl Ferdinand Cori, 51 (5 December 1896, Prague, Austria-Hungary (now Czech Republic, after Czechoslovakia) - 20 October 1984, Cambridge, MA, USA, aged 87.9), Czech-born American Professor at Washington University, St. Louis, MO, USA, and Gerty Theresa Cori, née Radnitz, 51 (5 December 1896, Prague, Austria-Hungary (now Czech Republic, after Czechoslovakia) - 26 October 1957, St. Louis, MO, USA, aged 61.1), Czech-born American Professor at Washington University, St. Louis, MO, USA, "for their discovery of the course of the catalytic conversion of glycogen", Bernardo Alberto Houssay, 60 ("for his discovery of the part played by the hormone of the anterior pituitary lobe in the metabolism of sugar".

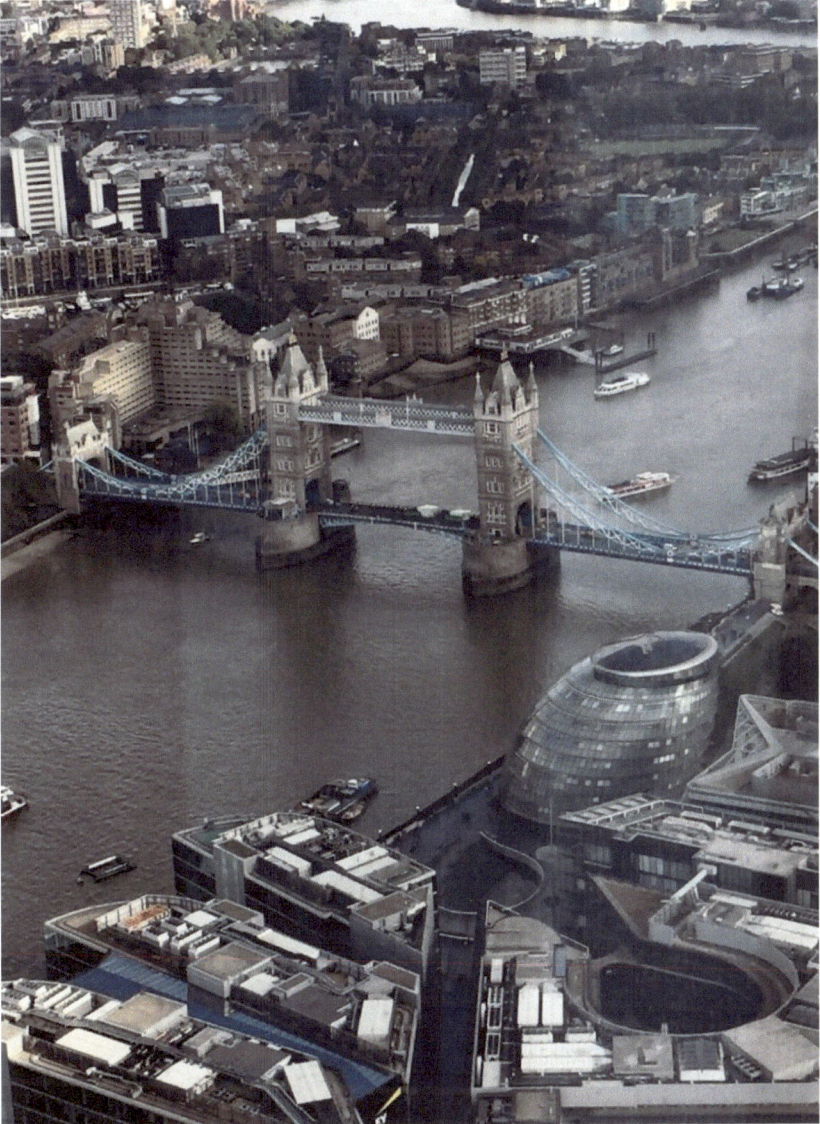

London, from the Shard (2012, 309 m, observatory at 244 m), looking east to the Tower Bridge (1886-1894, combined bascule and suspension turreted bridge over River Thames (flowing from west (left) to east (right)), between London boroughs Tower Hamlets (north – left up) and Southwark (south – right), length 244 m, height 65 m, longest span 82 m, clearance 8 m (closed), 42 m (open)), City Hall (2002, height 45 m, center right round, for the Greater London Authority: Mayor of London and the London Assembly)

1948 – Garrod, Macewen, Müller

- 22 June – 100th anniversary of the birth of **William Macewen** (22 June 1848 – 22 March 1924, aged 75 years and 9 months), Scottish surgeon.

- 100 years ago, in 1848, **Alfred Baring Garrod**, 29, (3 May 1819 – 28 December 1907, aged 88.6, English physician), observed that excess uric acid in the blood is the cause of gout.

- The Nobel Prize in Physiology or Medicine 1948 was awarded to **Paul Hermann Müller**, 49 (12 January 1899, Olten, Switzerland - 12 October 1965, Basel, Switzerland, aged 66 years and 9 months), Swiss Researcher at Laboratorium der Farben-Fabriken J.R. Geigy A.G. (Laboratory of the J.R. Geigy Dye-Factory Co.), Basel, Switzerland for his discovery in 1942 of the high efficiency of dichlorodiphenyltrichloroethane (DDT) as a contact poison against several arthropods, like mosquitoes, which spread malaria. With the aid of DDT, people could curb the spread of malaria, and halt an epidemic of typhus.

1949 – Jenner, Burnet, Hess, Moniz

- 17 May – 200th anniversary of the birth of **Edward Jenner** (17 May 1749, Berkeley, Gloucestershire, England – 26 Jan 1823, Berkeley, Gloucestershire, England, aged 73.6), English physician, surgeon and scientist, who, in 1796, at age 47, developed the process of vaccination for smallpox, the first vaccines for any disease. The terms "vaccine" and "vaccination" are derived from Variolae vaccinae, the term devised by Jenner to denote cowpox

- 100 years ago, in 1849, the safety pin was invented.

- Our immune system protects us against attacks by microorganisms, and rejects foreign tissue. Part of our immunity has a hereditary basis, but part of it is acquired, and is not present in the fetus. In 1949 **Macfarlane Burnet**, 50, theorized that the ability to distinguish between one's own, and foreign tissue, is not hereditary, but is acquired during the fetus stage.

- The Nobel Prize in Physiology or Medicine 1949 was awarded to **Walter Rudolf Hess**, 68 (17 March 1881, Frauenfeld, Switzerland - 12 August 1973, Ascona, Switzerland, aged 92.4), Swiss Professor at University of Zurich, Zurich, Switzerland, "for his discovery of the functional organization of the interbrain as a coordinator of the activities of the internal organs", and Antonio Caetano de Abreu Freire **Egas Moniz**, 75 (29 November 1874, Avanca, Portugal - 13 December 1955, Lisbon, Portugal, aged 81), Portuguese Professor at University of Lisbon, Lisbon, Portugal, Neurological Institute, Lisbon, Portugal, "for his discovery of the therapeutic value of leucotomy in certain psychoses".

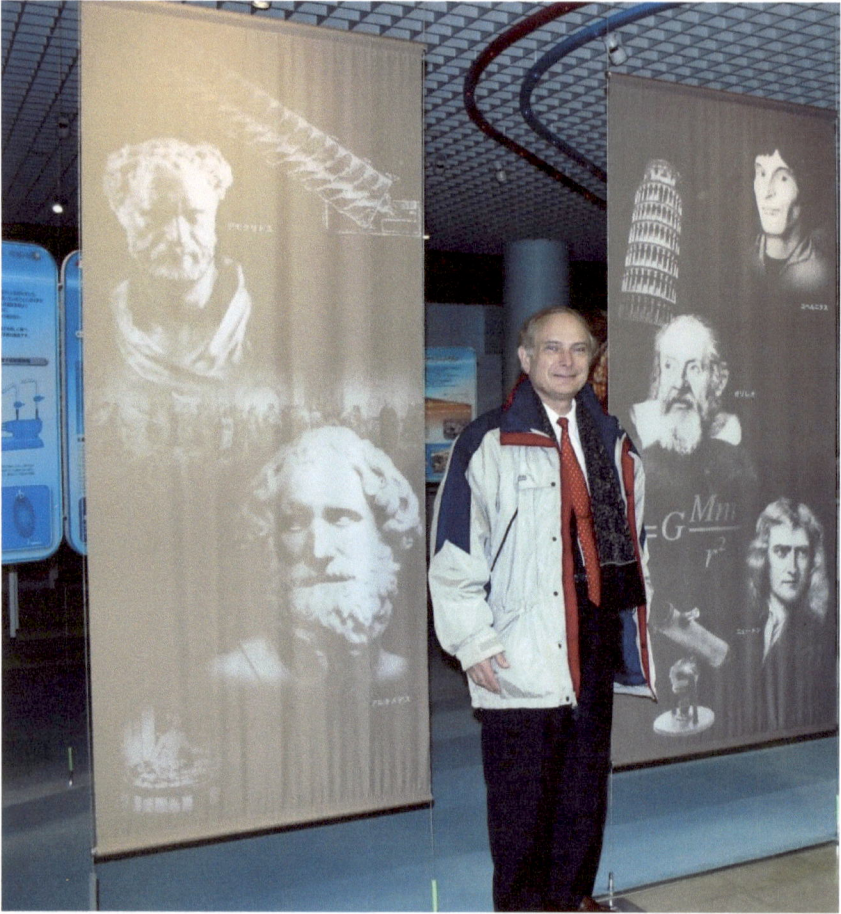

Japan, Tsukuba: 20 Nov 2008, inside the main research building, photographs with celebrity physicists, like Galileo Galilei (1564 – 1642, who used the Leaning Tower of Pisa, Italy (1173 – 1372), center-right), at the High Energy Accelerator Research Organization (KEK, 1997) in Tsukuba Science City (1962), in Ibaraki Prefecture, 60 km north-east of Tokyo.

1950 – Diocles of Carystus, Kendall, Hench, Hopps

- c. 2300 years ago, in 350 BC, **Diocles of Carystus** (in Latin Diocles Medicus, c. 400 BC, Carystus (on the south end of the Greek island of Euboea, facing the East Coast of Attica) – 320 BC, aged 80, philosopher and pioneer in medicine, second only to Hippocrates in reputation and ability) worked in Athens, and wrote the first known anatomy book.

- The Nobel Prize in Physiology or Medicine 1950 was awarded to **Edward Calvin Kendall**, 64 (8 March 1886, South Norwalk, CT, USA - 4 May 1972, Princeton, NJ, USA, aged 86.1), American Researcher at Mayo Clinic, Rochester, MN, USA, **Tadeus Reichstein,** 53 (20 July 1897, Wloclawek, Poland - 1 August 1996, Basel, Switzerland, aged 99 years and 12 days), Polish-born Swiss Professor at Basel University, Basel, Switzerland, and **Philip Showalter Hench**, 54 (28 February 1896, Pittsburgh, PA, USA - 30 March 1965, Ocho Rios, Jamaica, aged 69.1), American Professor at Mayo Clinic, Rochester, MN, USA "for their discoveries relating to the hormones of the adrenal cortex, their structure and biological effects".

- **John Alexander Hopps**, 31 (21 May 1919, Winnipeg, Canada – 24 November 1998, aged 79.5), Canadian engineer invented the first cardiac pacemaker.

1951 – **Bond, Theiler, Medawar**

- 11 May – 200 years ago, in 1751, Pennsylvania Hospital was founded in Philadelphia by Benjamin Franklin, 45, and **Thomas Bond**, 37, (2 May 1713 – 26 March 1784, aged 70.9, American physician and surgeon).

- 14 June – the computer UNIVAC I is dedicated by the U.S. Census Bureau.

- **Max Theiler**, 52 (30 January 1899, Pretoria, South Africa - 11 August 1972, New Haven, CT, USA, aged 73.6), of the Rockefeller Foundation (Laboratories of the Division of Medicine and Public Health, Rockefeller Foundation, New York, NY, USA), was awarded the Nobel Prize in Physiology or Medicine 1951, for developing a vaccine (17D) against yellow fever in 1937, at age 38.

- **Peter Medawar** (the Nobel Prize in Physiology or Medicine 1960) successfully transplanted tissue between mouse fetuses without rejection in 1951. He could perform new transplants on the mice when they became adults, something that did not work when the transplants were not performed during the fetus stage. The results had significance for organ transplants.

1952 – da Vinci, Waksman, Zoll, Salk

– 15 April – 500th anniversary of the birth of **Leonardo da Vinci** (full name Leonardo di ser Piero da Vinci, 15 April 1452, Anchiano near Vinci (25 km west of Florence, on a Tuscan hill, in the lower valley of the Arno River), Republic of Florence (ruled by de Medici) – 2 May 1519, Amboise, Kingdom of France, aged 67 years and 17 days), Italian polymath whose areas of interest included invention, painting, sculpting, architecture, science, music, mathematics, engineering, literature, anatomy, geology, astronomy, optics, botany, hydrodynamics, writing, history, and cartography, but he did not publish his findings. He is the father of paleontology, ichnology, and architecture, and is one of the greatest painters of all time. In 1487, Leonardo da Vinci, 35, drew L'Uomo Vitruviano (the Vitruvian Man, now at Accademia in Venice), which is regarded as a cultural icon, being reproduced on the euro coin, textbooks, etc. Vitruvius was an ancient Roman architect, interested in the proportions of the human body. In 1489 Leonardo da Vinci, 37, dissected for anatomical research, and he also painted Lady with an Ermine, the lady being Cecilia Gallerani – finished by 1490. In 1510, Leonardo, 58, collaborated with Professor doctor Marcantonio della Torre, 29, on his work of theoretical anatomy – until 1511, when Marcantonio della Torre died at the very young age of 30. In 1508 Leonardo da Vinci illustrated the concept of contact lenses.

.
- The Nobel Prize in Physiology or Medicine 1952 was awarded to **Selman A. Waksman**, 64 (22 July 1888, Priluka (now Nova Pryluka), Russian Empire (now Ukraine) - 16 August 1973, Hyannis, MA, USA, aged 85.) Russian-born, American professor, inventor, biochemist and microbiologist, who discovered at Rutgers University (New Brunswick, NJ, USA), in 1943 (age 55), the antibiotic streptomycin, he first antibiotic effective against tuberculosis.

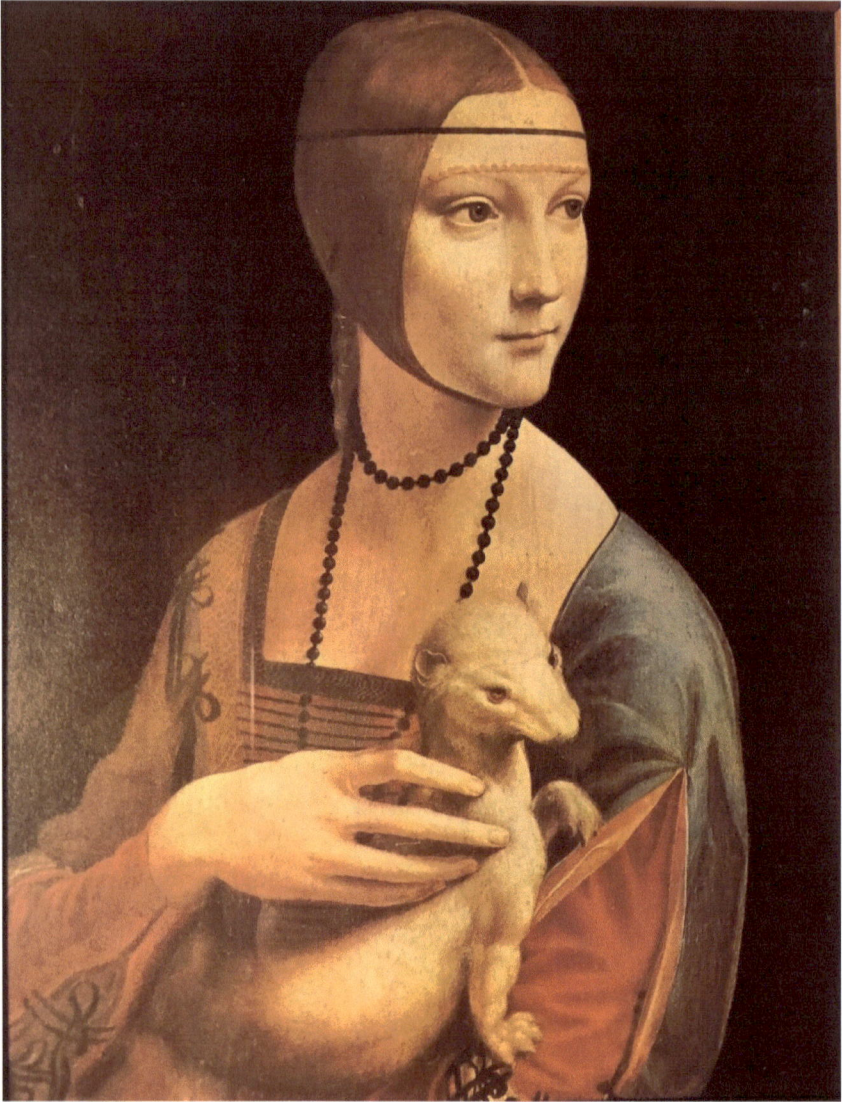

Leonardo da Vinci, 38, 1490, Lady with an Ermine (the lady being Cecilia Gallerani)

- By measuring changes in electrical charges in a very large nerve fiber from a species of octopus, **Alan Hodgkin** and **Andrew Huxley** (both received the Nobel Prize in 1963) were able to show how nerve impulses are exchanged between cells. In 1952 they could demonstrate that a fundamental mechanism involves the passage of sodium and potassium ions in opposite directions in and out through the cell wall, which gives rise to electrical charges.

In 1952 Andrew Huxley turned to muscle contraction, and developed an interference microscope for studying the striation pattern in isolated muscle fibers.

- **Paul Maurice Zoll**, 41 (15 July 1911, Boston, MA – 5 January 1999, Newton, MA, aged 87.5), American cardiologist and one of the pioneers in the development of the artificial cardiac pacemaker and cardiac defibrillator. He graduated from Boston Latin School in 1928, and from Harvard College in 1936.

- **Jonas Edward Salk**, 36 (28 October 1914, New York City, NY – 23 June 1995, La Jolla, CA, aged 80.6), American medical researcher and virologist, who discovered and developed one of the first successful polio vaccines.

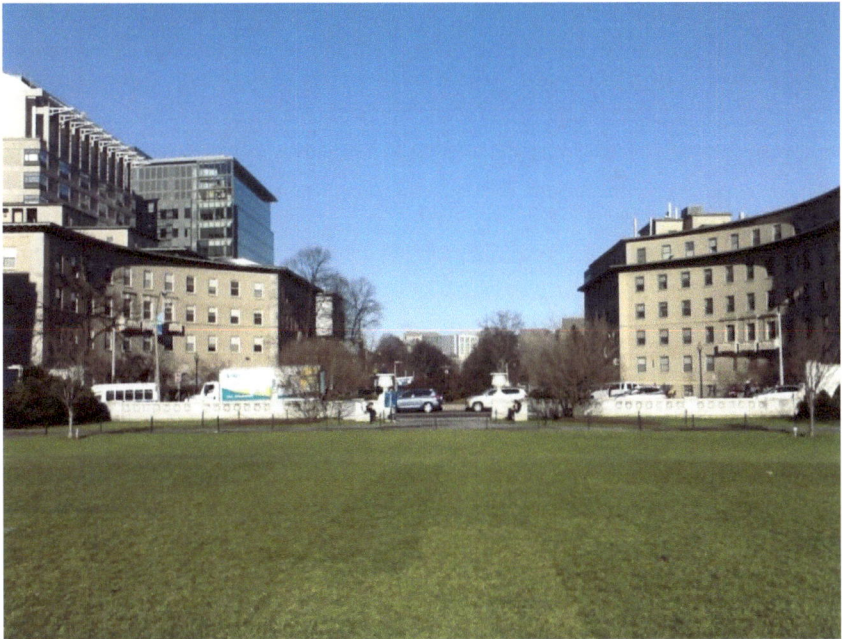

Boston: 3 Dec 2009, from Harvard Medical School looking northeast to the Avenue Louis Pasteur (1822-1895, French microbiologist),

Chapter 2. 1953 – 1962: Pylarini, Amyand, Pasteur, Palade

1953 – Crick, Watson, Krebs, Lipmann

- **Francis Crick**, 37 (8 June 1916, Weston Favell, Northampton, United Kingdom – 28 July 2004, University of California San Diego, San Diego, CA, aged 88.1, British molecular biologist, biophysicist, and neuroscientist, who, in 1953, co-authored with James Watson the academic paper proposing the double helix structure of the DNA molecule) and **James Watson**, 25 (born: April 6, 1928 (now over the age of 90 years), Chicago, IL, American molecular biologist, geneticist and zoologist.) determined the structure of the DNA molecule. This structure - a long double helix - contains a long row of pairs of four different nitrogen bases, which allow the molecule to function like a code. The molecule's structure also explains how it is able to copy itself. The nitrogen bases always pair in the same constellations, so that if a molecule is split, its halves can be supplemented, so that they form copies of the original molecule. They received the Nobel Prize in Physiology or Medicine 1962, with **Maurice Hugh Frederick Wilkins.**

- The Nobel Prize in Physiology or Medicine 1953 was awarded to **Hans Adolf Krebs**, 53 (25 August 1900, Hildesheim, Germany - 22 November 1981, Oxford, United Kingdom, aged 81.2), German-born British Professor at Sheffield University, Sheffield, United Kingdom, "for his discovery of the citric acid cycle", and **Fritz Albert Lipmann**, 54 (12 June 1899, Koenigsberg (now Kaliningrad), Germany (now Russia) - 24 July 1986, Poughkeepsie, NY, USA, aged 87.1), German-born American Professor at Harvard Medical School, Boston, MA, USA, Massachusetts General Hospital, Boston, MA, USA, "for his discovery of co-enzyme A and its importance for intermediary metabolism".

1954 – von Behring, Enders, Weller, Robbins, Murray

- 14 March - 100th anniversary of the birth of **Paul Ehrlich** (14 March 1854, Strehlen, Silesia, Prussia (now Strzelin, Poland) – 20 Aug. 1915, Bad Homburg vor der Höhe, Germany, aged 61.4) was a Nobel prize-winning German physician and scientist (a member of Koch's research team) who worked in the fields of hematology, immunology, and antimicrobial chemotherapy. He is credited with finding a cure for syphilis in 1909.

- 15 March - 100th anniversary of the birth of **Emil von Behring**, born as Emil Adolf Behring (15 March 1854, Hansdorf, Prussia (now Lawice, Poland) – 31 March 1917, Marburg, Germany, aged 63 years and 16 days), German physiologist who received, at 47, the 1901 Nobel Prize in Physiology or Medicine, the first one awarded, for his discovery of a diphtheria antitoxin. He was widely known as a "savior of children," as diphtheria used to be a major cause of child death. In 1890 Emil von Behring, 36, discovered antitoxins, and developed tetanus and diphtheria vaccines.

- The Nobel Prize in Physiology or Medicine 1954 was awarded to **John Franklin Enders**, 57 (10 February 1897, West Hartford, CT, USA - 8 September 1985, Waterford, CT, USA, aged 88.6), American Professor at Harvard Medical School, Boston, MA, USA, Research Division of Infectious Diseases, Children's Medical Center, Boston, MA, USA, **Thomas Huckle Weller**, 39 (15 June 1915, Ann Arbor, MI, USA - 23 August 2008, Needham, MA, USA, aged 93.2), American Researcher at Research Division of Infectious Diseases, Children's Medical Center, Boston, MA, USA, and **Frederick Chapman Robbins**, 38 (25 August 1916, Auburn, AL, USA - 4 August 2003, Cleveland, OH, USA, aged 86.9), American Professor at Western Reserve University, Cleveland, OH, USA, "for their discovery of the ability of poliomyelitis viruses to grow in cultures of various types of tissue".

- 23 December - **Joseph Edward Murray**, 35.7 (1 April 1919, Milford, MA – 26 November 2012, Boston, MA, aged 93 years 7 months and 25 days; he had six children), American plastic surgeon, performed the first successful human kidney transplant on identical twins.

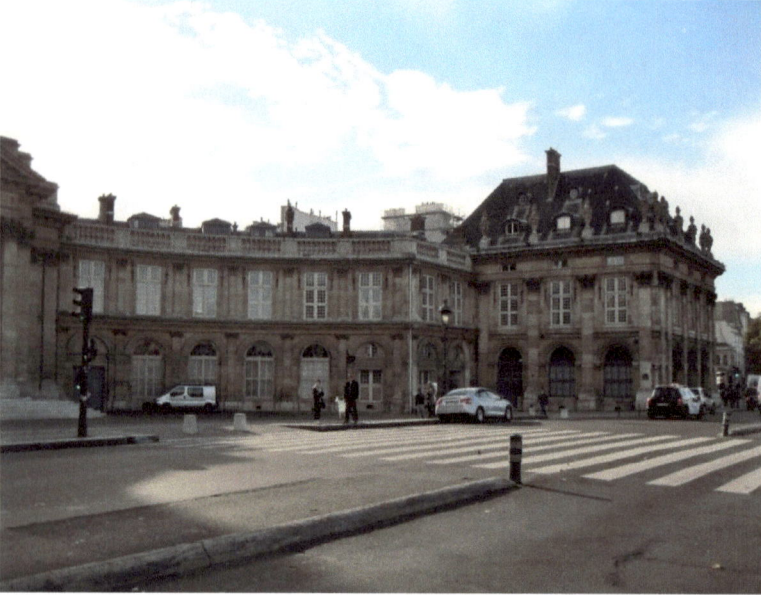

France, Paris, the north-west part of L'Institut de France (1795, moved in 1805 by Napoléon in this baroque building from 1684) is a revered French cultural society with five académies, the most famous being Académie Français (1635) and. Académie des sciences (1666).

1955 – Mellanby, Palade, Theorell

- 30 January - Sir **Edward Mellanby,** British physician, physiologist, pharmacologist, and nutrition scientist, passed away at the age of 70.8 (8 April 1884, West Hartlepool, United Kingdom – 30 Jan 1955, Mill Hill, London, United Kingdom). He discovered vitamin D, and its role in preventing rickets, in 1919, at age 35, working at King's College for Women, in London. In 1921, Edward Mellanby, 37, discovered that lack of vitamin D in the diet causes osteomalacia (rickets).

- 11 March - Sir **Alexander Fleming,** British physician, microbiologist, and pharmacologist, passed away at the age of 73.6 (6 Aug 1881, Darvel, UK – 11 March 1955, London, UK). His best-known discoveries are the enzyme lysozyme in 1923 (age 42), and in 1928 (age 47) penicillin - the world's first antibiotic substance. He received the Nobel Prize in Physiology or Medicine in 1945, at age 64, with Howard Florey and Ernst Boris Chain.

- **George Palade,** 43, discovered previously unknown organelles in the cell, ribosomes, where the cell's formation of proteins takes place. He also identified the paths proteins take through the cell. He received the Nobel Prize in 1974.

- The Nobel Prize in Physiology or Medicine 1955 was awarded to **Axel Hugo Theodor Theorell**, 52 (6 July 1903, Linköping, Sweden - 15 August 1982, Stockholm, Sweden, aged 79.1), Swedish Professor at Karolinska Institutet, Nobel Medical Institute, Stockholm, Sweden, "for his discoveries concerning the nature and mode of action of oxidation enzymes".

1956 – **Plummer**, **Kornberg, Cournand, Forssmann, Richards**

- 16 April – 200 years ago, in 1756, **Andrew Plummer**, Scottish physician and chemist, died at the age of 59 (1697–1756).

- By studying bacteria, **Arthur Kornberg** succeeded in isolating DNA polymerase in 1956 - an enzyme that is active in the formation of DNA. Using a DNA molecule as a blueprint, the enzyme builds a copy of the DNA molecule from nucleotides, which are the building blocks of DNA.

- The Nobel Prize in Physiology or Medicine 1956 was awarded to **André Frédéric Cournand**, 61 (24 September 1895, Paris, France - 19 February 1988, Great Barrington, MA, USA, aged 92.4), French-born American Professor at Columbia University Division, Cardio-Pulmonary Laboratory, Bellevue Hospital, New York, NY, USA, **Werner Forssmann**, 52 (29 August 1904, Berlin, Germany - 1 June 1979, Schopfheim, West Germany (now Germany), aged 74.7; had six children), German Professor at Mainz University, Mainz, Federal Republic of Germany, Bad Kreuznach, Federal Republic of Germany, and **Dickinson W. Richards**, 61 (30 October 1895, Orange, NJ, USA - 23 February 1973, Lakeville, CT, USA, aged 77.3), American Professor at Columbia University, New York, NY, USA, "for their discoveries concerning heart catheterization and pathological changes in the circulatory system".

1957 – Huygens, Pasteur, Weigl, Bovet,

- 300 years ago, in 1657, **Christiaan Huygens**, 28, (14 April 1629 – 8 July 1695, aged 66.2, Dutch mathematician, physicist, astronomer and inventor) developed the first functional pendulum clock, based on the learnings of Galileo Galilei, and became the most accurate timekeeper for almost 270 years, and it is still in use.

- 100 years ago, in 1857, **Louis Pasteur**, 35, identified germs as clause of disease.

- 11 August - **Rudolf Stefan Weigl**, Polish biologist and inventor, passed away at the age of 73.9 (2 September 1883, Prerau, Austria-Hungary – 11 August 1957, Zakopane, Poland). He discovered in 1933 (age 50) the first effective vaccine against epidemic typhus.

- The Nobel Prize in Physiology or Medicine 1957 was awarded to **Daniel Bovet**, 50 (23 March 1907, Neuchâtel, Switzerland - 8 April 1992, Rome, Italy, aged 85), Swiss-born Italian Researcher at Istituto Superiore di Sanità (Chief Institute of Public Health), Rome, Italy, "for his discoveries relating to synthetic compounds that inhibit the action of certain body substances, and especially their action on the vascular system and the skeletal muscles".

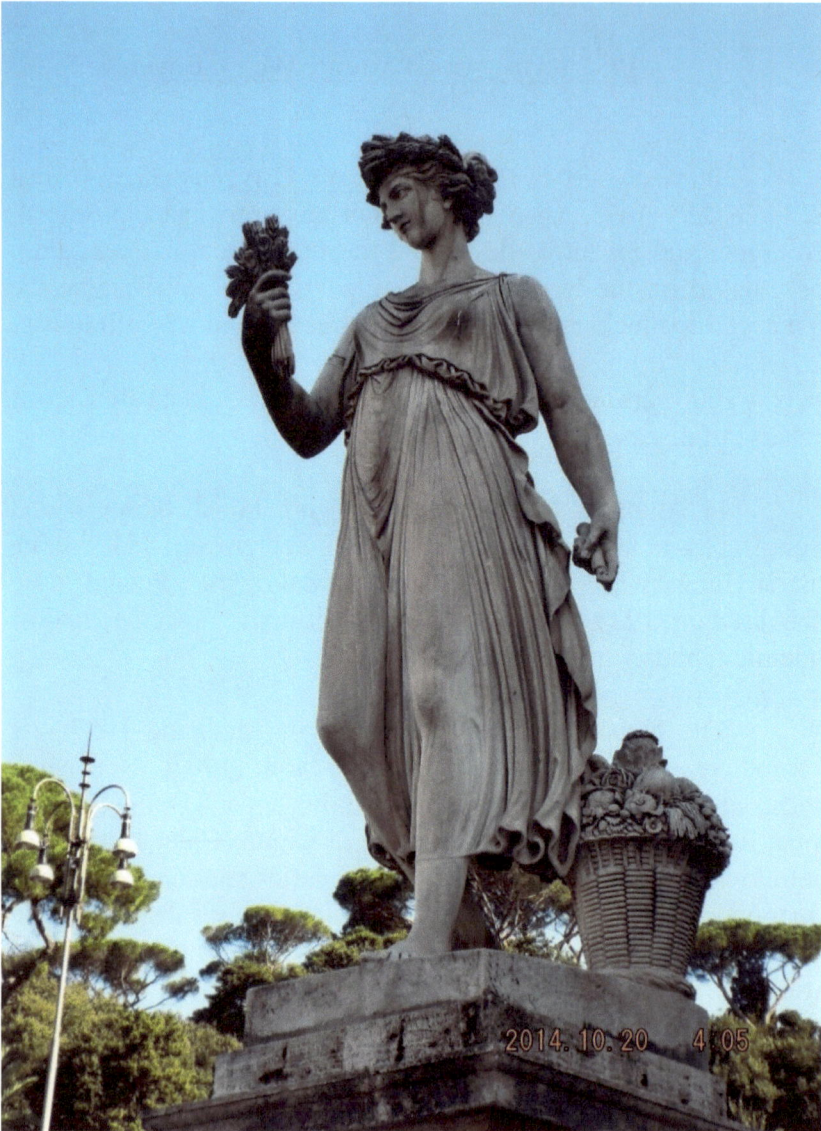

Italy, Roma (753 BC, one of the oldest occupied cities in Europe, called Roma Aeterna (The Eternal City) and Caput Mundi (Capital of the World)), southeast of Piazza del Popolo (1822, by Giuseppe Valadier, inside the northern gate in the Aurelian Walls, the Porta Flaminia, now called the Porta del Popolo), near Via del Babuino (opened in 1525 as the Via Paolina) and the church Santa Maria in Montesanto (1679, begun by Rainaldi and completed by Bernini and Fontana), the statue of the Goddess of Abundance.

1958 – Sachs, Bouchut, Beadle, Tatum, Lederberg

- 2 January - 100th anniversary of the birth of **Bernard Sachs** (2 January 1858 – 8 February 1944, aged 86.1), American neurologist.

- 100 years ago, in 1858, French pediatrician **Eugène Bouchut**, 40, (18 May 1818 – 26 November 1891, aged 73.5, French physician who made important contributions in pediatrics, laryngology, neurology and ophthalmology), developed a new technique for non-surgical orotracheal intubation to bypass laryngeal obstruction resulting from a diphtheria-related pseudomembrane.

- The Nobel Prize in Physiology or Medicine 1958 was awarded to **George Wells Beadle**, 55 (22 October 1903, Wahoo, NE, USA - 9 June 1989, Pomona, CA, USA, aged 85.6), American Professor at California Institute of Technology (Caltech), Pasadena, CA, USA, and **Edward Lawrie Tatum**, 49 (14 December 1909, Boulder, CO, USA - 5 November 1975, New York, NY, USA, aged 65.9), "for their discovery that genes act by regulating definite chemical events", and **Joshua Lederberg**, 33 (23 May 1925, Montclair, NJ, USA - 2 February 2008, New York, NY, USA, aged 82.7), American Professor at University of Wisconsin, Madison, WI, USA, "for his discoveries concerning genetic recombination and the organization of the genetic material of bacteria".

1959 – Pylarini, Mosse, Ochoa, Kornberg

- 9 January – 300th anniversary of the birth of **Giacomo Pylarini** (9 Jan 1659, Cephalonia, Greece – 1718, Padua, Italy, aged 59), Venetian physician and consul for the Republic of Venice in Smyrna (Greek city from antiquity, located at a central point on the Aegean coast of Anatolia; after 1930 the name was changed to İzmir, in Turkey), who in 1701, at the age of 42, on the children of the English ambassador to Constantinople, gave the first smallpox inoculation outside of Asia. This early immunization effort was called "variolation".

- 16 February – 200 years ago, in 1759, **Bartholomew Mosse**, Irish surgeon, and impresario responsible for founding the Rotunda Hospital in Dublin, died at the age of 47 (1712 – 16 February 1759).

- The Nobel Prize in Physiology or Medicine 1959 was awarded to **Severo Ochoa**, 54 (24 September 1905, Luarca, Spain - 1 November 1993, Madrid, Spain, aged 88.1), Spanish-born American Professor at New York University, College of Medicine, New York, NY, USA, and **Arthur Kornberg**, 41 (3 March 1918, Brooklyn, NY, USA - 26 October 2007, Stanford, CA, USA, aged 89.6), American Professor at Stanford University, Stanford, CA, USA, "for their discovery of the mechanisms in the biological synthesis of ribonucleic acid and deoxyribonucleic acid".

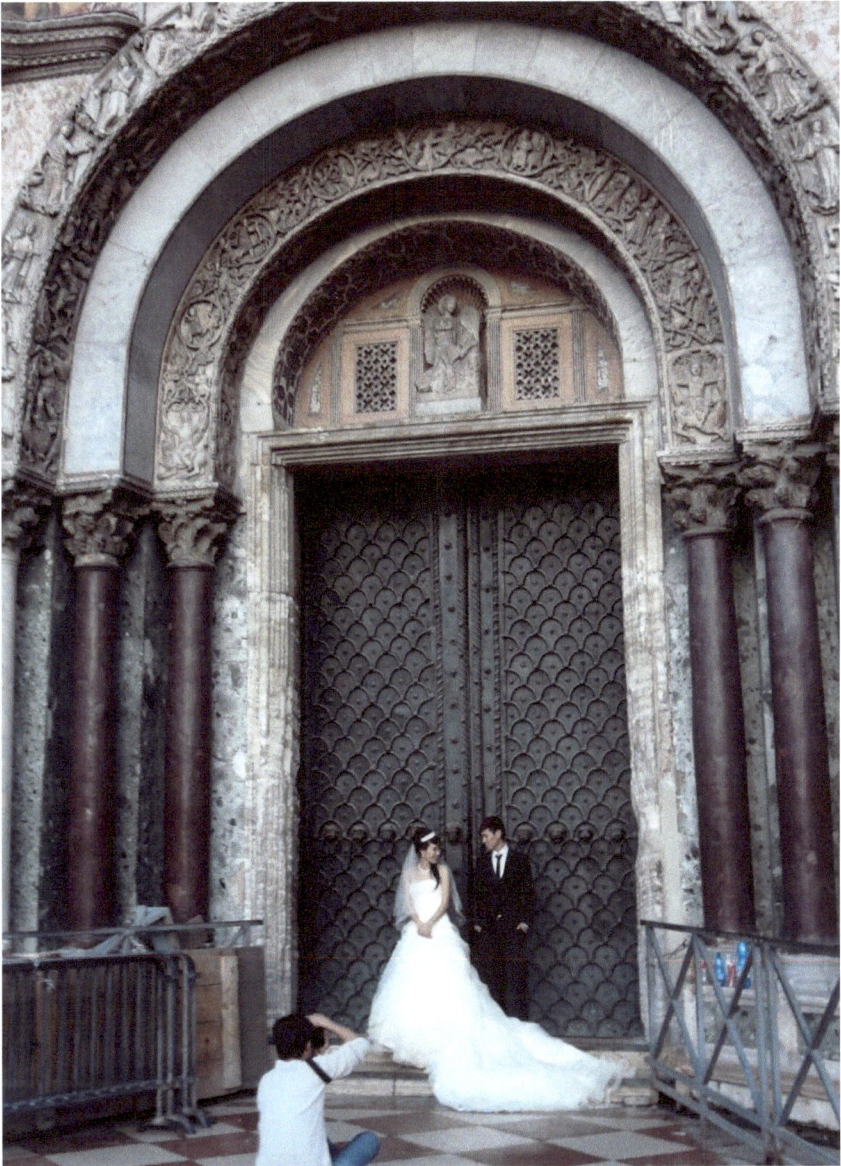

Italy, Venezia: In the middle of the west façade of the Basilica di San Marco, we see the central bronze-fashioned door, in a round-arched portal, encircled by polychrome marble columns. Above this door there are three round bas-relief cycles of Romanesque art. A Japanese couple, with their Japanese photographer, make their wedding photographs in this most beautiful place.

1960 – Amyand, Haffkine, Burnet, Medawar

- 300th anniversary of the birth of **Claudius Amyand** (1660, Mornac, Saintonge, France – 6 July 1740, London, UK, aged 80), French born surgeon, who performed the first recorded successful appendectomy. As Huguenots, the Amyands fled to England following the revocation of the Edict of Nantes in 1685, when Claudius was 25, and settled in London. At St. George's Hospital, on 6 December 1735, he (age 75) performed the first recorded successful appendicectomy (which is the surgical removal of the vermiform appendix). The patient was an 11-year boy named Hanvil Anderson, who had an inguinal hernia combined with an acutely inflamed appendix. This situation, where the appendix is included in the hernial sac, is known as an Amyand's hernia. Amyand described the operation himself in a paper for the Royal Society.

- 100th anniversary of the birth of Sir **Waldemar Haffkine** (born Vladimir Aronovich Havkin, 15 March 1860; Berdyansk, Russian Empire – 26 October 1930, Lausanne, Switzerland, aged 70.6), Russian bacteriologist who, in 1897, at age 37, developed the first vaccine for bubonic plague, and did prophylactic vaccination against cholera and bubonic plague in British India.

- The Nobel Prize in Physiology or Medicine 1960 was awarded to Sir **Frank Macfarlane Burnet**, 61 (3 September 1899, Traralgon, Australia - 31 August 1985, Melbourne, Australia, aged 85.99, just 3 days before 86), Australian Professor at Walter and Eliza Hall Institute for Medical Research, Melbourne, Australia, and **Peter Brian Medawar**, 45 (28 February 1915, Rio de Janeiro, Brazil - 2 October 1987, London, United Kingdom, aged 72.6), Brazilian-born British Professor at University College, London, United Kingdom, "for discovery of acquired immunological tolerance".

1961 – Ménière, Broca, Dickson, Békésy

- 100 years ago, in 1861:

- **Prosper Ménière**, 62, (18 June 1799 – 7 February 1862, aged 62.6, French doctor who first identified a medical condition combining vertigo, hearing loss and tinnitus, which is now known as Ménière's disease), presented the association of vertigo with inner ear disorders.

- **Adolf Zsigmondy**, 45, (24 April 1816 – 23 June 1880, aged 64.1, dentist who lived in Vienna), developed a dental notation system.

- **Paul Broca**, 37, (28 June 1824 – 9 July 1880, aged 56 years and 11 days, French physician, anatomist and anthropologist), identified the speech production center of the brain.

21 September - **Earle Dickson,** American inventor, passed away at the age of 68.9 (10 Oct 1892, Tennessee, USA – 21 Sep 1961, Kitchener, Canada). He is best known for creating in 1921, at age 29, Band-Aid® brand adhesive bandages, at the Johnson & Johnson Company, where he served as Vice President.

- The Nobel Prize in Physiology or Medicine 1961 was awarded to **Georg von Békésy**, 62 (3 June 1899, Budapest, Hungary - 13 June 1972, Honolulu, HI, USA, aged 73 years and 10 days), Hungarian-born American Professor at Harvard University, Cambridge, MA, USA, "for his discoveries of the physical mechanism of stimulation within the cochlea".

1962 – Snellen, Raynaud, Crick, Watson, Wilkins

- 100 years ago, in 1862, **Hermann Snellen**, 28, (19 February 1834 – January 18, 1908, aged 73.9, Dutch ophthalmologist), published the Snellen chart for testing visual acuity.

- 100 years ago, in 1862, **Maurice Raynaud**, 28, (10 August 1834 – 29 June 1881, aged 46.9, French doctor), discovered Raynaud syndrome, a vasospastic disorder which contracts blood vessels in extremities. Snellen was 5 months and 22 days older than Raynaud, and died 26.5 years after Raynaud.

- The Nobel Prize in Physiology or Medicine 1962 was awarded to **Francis Harry Compton Crick**, 46 (8 June 1916, Northampton, United Kingdom - 28 July 2004, San Diego, CA, USA, aged 88.1), British Researcher at MRC Laboratory of Molecular Biology, Cambridge, United Kingdom, **James Dewey Watson**, 34 (born: 6 April 1928, Chicago, IL, USA), American Professor at Harvard University, Cambridge, MA, USA, and **Maurice Hugh Frederick Wilkins**, 46 (15 December 1916, Pongaroa, New Zealand - 5 October 2004, London, United Kingdom, aged 87.8), New Zealander-born British Professor at London University, London, United Kingdom, "for their discoveries concerning the molecular structure of nucleic acids and its significance for information transfer in living material".

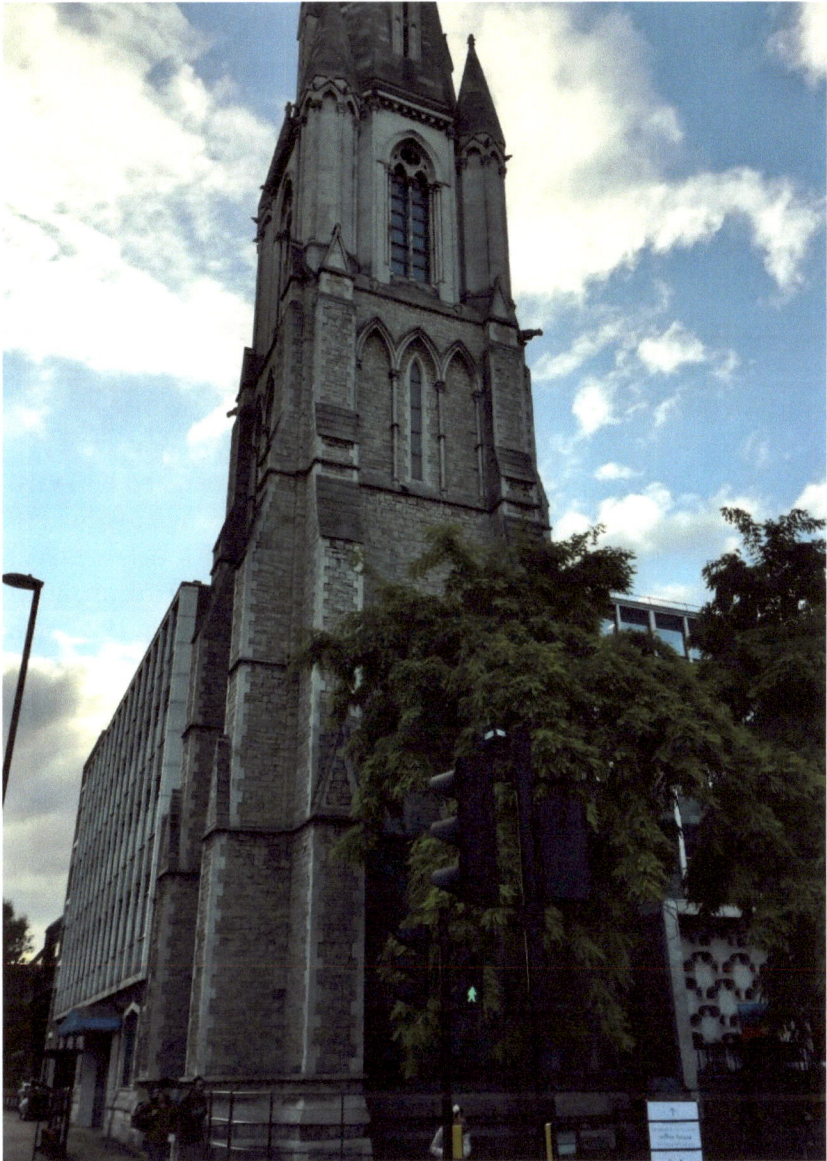

London: From Kennington Road (to right) at Westminster Bridge Road (left), looking southeast to Oasis Academy, South Bank (left down), and Oasis Church Waterloo (1783, 1985, Baptist). Just 50 m south (to left) of Lambeth North Station (for the underground Waterloo line, between Elephant & Castle and Waterloo), 500 m south from the Waterloo Station (for trains and for subway), and 1 km southeast from the Westminster Bridge.

Chapter 3. 1963 – 1972: Herophilus, Galenus, Hooke, Alzheimer, Barnard

1963 – Hooke, Ramon, Eccles, Hodgkin, Huxley, Enders

- 300 years ago, in 1663, **Robert Hooke**, 28, (28 July 1635 – 3 March 1703, aged 67.6) discovered cells using a microscope.

- 100 years ago, in 1863 - Formation of the **International Red Cross,** which was followed by the adoption of the First Geneva Convention in 1864.

- 8 June - **Gaston Ramon,** French veterinarian and biologist at the Pasteur Institute in France, passed away at the age of 76.7 (30 Sep 1886, Bellechaume, France – 8 June 1963 of a heart attack, Paris, France). He is best known for his role in the treatment of diphtheria and tetanus, and developed diphtheria toxoid in 1923 (age 37), the first vaccine for diphtheria. In 1923, Alexander Glenny perfected a method to inactivate tetanus toxin with formaldehyde. The same method was used to develop a vaccine against diphtheria in 1926. Pertussis (whooping cough) vaccine development took considerably longer, with a whole cell vaccine first licensed for use in the US in 1948.

- The Nobel Prize in Physiology or Medicine 1963 was awarded to Sir **John Carew Eccles**, 60 (27 January 1903, Melbourne, Australia - 2 May 1997, Contra, Switzerland, aged 94.3; he had nine children), Australian Professor at Australian National University, Canberra, Australia, **Alan Lloyd Hodgkin**, 49 (5 February 1914, Banbury, United Kingdom - 20 December 1998, Cambridge, United Kingdom, aged 84.8), British Professor at University of Cambridge, Cambridge, United Kingdom, and **Andrew Fielding Huxley**, 46 (22 November 1917, Hampstead, United Kingdom - 30 May 2012, Grantchester, United Kingdom, aged 94.5; he had six children), British Professor at University College, London, United Kingdom, "for their discoveries concerning the ionic mechanisms involved in excitation and inhibition in the peripheral and central portions of the nerve cell membrane".

- **Thomas J. Fogarty**, 29, (born 25 February 1934 (now age 85 years), Cincinnati, OH), American surgeon and medical device inventor, who invented the balloon embolectomy catheter, which improved the treatment of blood clots.

- **John Franklin Enders**, 68 (10 February 1897, West Hartford, CT, USA - 8 September 1985, Waterford, CT, USA, aged 88.6, American Professor at Harvard Medical School, Boston, MA, USA, Research Division of Infectious Diseases, Children's Medical Center, Boston, MA, USA), and colleagues transformed their Edmonston-B strain of measles virus into a vaccine, and licensed it in the United States.

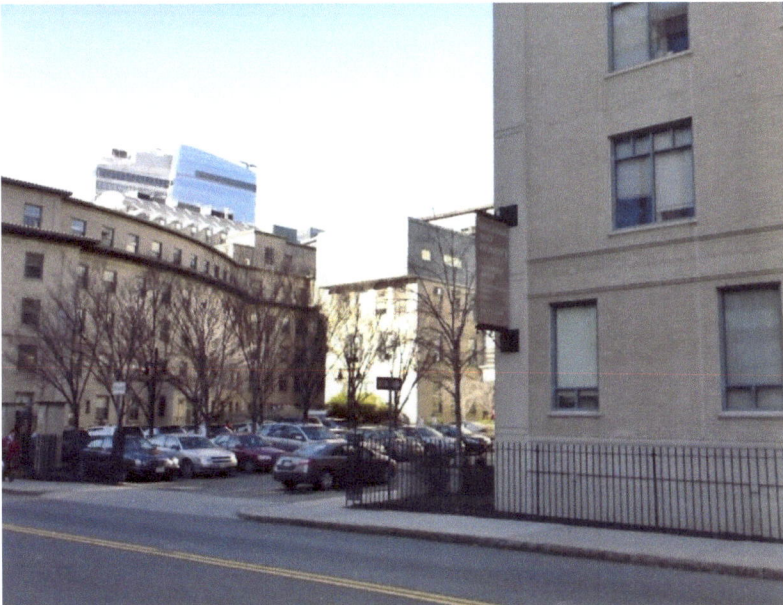

USA, Boston: 3 Dec 2009, Brigham and Women's Hospital (1980, three old hospitals merged) at 221 Longwood Avenue (right).

1964 – Galilei, Kraepelin, Alzheimer, Bloch, Lynen

- 15 February - 400th anniversary of the birth of **Galileo Galilei** (15 February 1564 – 8 January 1642, aged 77.9), Italian polymath. Known for his work as mathematician, astronomer, physicist, engineer, and philosopher, Galileo has been called the "father of observational astronomy", the "father of modern physics", the "father of the scientific method", and the "father of science".

- 14 June - 100th anniversary of the birth of **Aloysius Alzheimer** (14 June 1864 – 19 December 1915, aged 51.5), German psychiatrist and neuropathologist, colleague of **Emil Kraepelin**, 8.3, (15 February 1856 – 7 October 1926, aged 70.6, had 8 children, German psychiatrist, founder of modern scientific psychiatry, psychopharmacology and psychiatric genetics). Alzheimer identified the first published case, on 3 Nov 1906 (age 42.4), of "presenile dementia", which Kraepelin would later, in 1910 (age 46), call as Alzheimer's disease.

- The Nobel Prize in Physiology or Medicine 1964 was awarded to **Konrad Bloch**, 52 (21 January 1912, Neisse (now Nysa), Germany (now Poland) - 15 October 2000, Burlington, MA, USA, aged 88.7), German-born American Professor at Harvard University, Cambridge, MA, USA, and **Feodor Lynen**, 53 (6 April 1911, Munich, Germany - 6 August 1979, Munich, Germany, aged 68 years and 4 months), German Professor at Max-Planck-Institut für Zellchemie, Munich, Federal Republic of Germany, "for their discoveries concerning the mechanism and regulation of the cholesterol and fatty acid metabolism".

1965 – Herophilus, Schultze, Jacob, Lwoff, Monod

- 2300th anniversary of the birth of **Herophilus** (or Herophilos, c. 335 BC, Chalcedon, Bithynia, Greece – 280 BC, Alexandria, Egypt, aged 55, Greek physician, the father of anatomy, spent the majority of his life in Alexandria. He was the first scientist to systematically perform scientific dissections, and he studied the nervous system.

- 100 years ago, in 1865, **Louis Pasteur**, 43, (27 December 1822, Dole, France – 28 September 1895, Marnes-la-Coquette, France, aged 72.7, French biologist, microbiologist and chemist), shows that the air is full of bacteria.

- 100 years ago, in 1865, **Max Schultze**, 40, (25 March 1825 – 16 January 1874, aged 48.8, German microscopic anatomist) presented the first description of the platelet.

- The Nobel Prize in Physiology or Medicine 1965 was awarded to **François Jacob**, 45 (17 June 1920, Nancy, France - 19 April 2013, Paris, France, aged 92.9), French Researcher at Institut Pasteur, Paris, France, **André Lwoff**, 63 (8 May 1902, Ainay-le-Château, France - 30 September 1994, Paris, France, aged 92.4), French Researcher at Institut Pasteur, Paris, France, and **Jacques Monod**, 55 (9 February 1910, Paris, France - 31 May 1976, Cannes, France, aged 66.3), French Researcher at Institut Pasteur, Paris, France, "for their discoveries concerning genetic control of enzyme and virus synthesis".

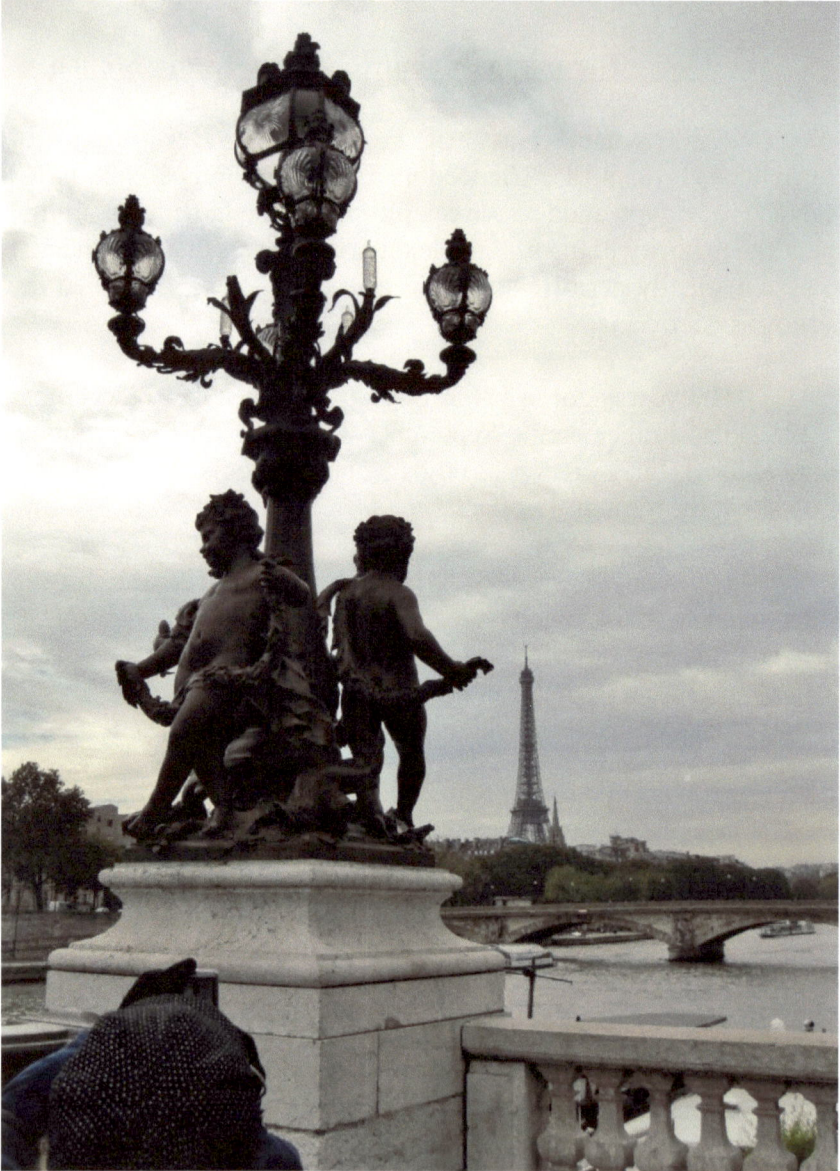

Paris: view (looking south-west) of nymph statues on an Art Nouveau lamp, on the west side of Pont Alexandre III (1896-1900, for Alexander III (1845-1894), Tsar of Russia, King of Poland and Grand Prince of Finland (1881-1894)), Pont des Invalides (center – right), and the north-east side of Tour Eiffel (1889, 324 m, 279 m at the 3rd level).

1966 – Despeignes, Allbutt, Rous, Huggins

- 14 February - 100th anniversary of the birth of **Victor Despeignes** (14 February 1866 – 30 July 1937, aged 71.4), French creator of radiation oncology. In July 1896, at age 30.4, he was the first physician to use X-rays to treat cancer, for a patient with stomach cancer. He was also the first physician to publish a paper on radiation therapy, in 1896, about that case. This attempt was less than a year after the publication of the discovery of X-rays by Wilhelm Röntgen. He became the chief of the laboratory of Louis Pasteur in 1892, at the age of 26.

- 100 years ago, in 1866, **Thomas Clifford Allbutt**, 30, (20 July 1836 – 22 February 1925, aged 88.6, English physician) invented a clinical thermometer. He was the president of the British Medical Association 1920.

- The Nobel Prize in Physiology or Medicine 1966 was awarded to **Peyton Rous**, 87 (5 October 1879, Baltimore, MD, USA - 16 February 1970, New York, NY, USA, aged 90.3), American Professor at Rockefeller University, New York, NY, USA, "for his discovery of tumor-inducing viruses", and **Charles Brenton Huggins,** 65 (22 September 1901, Halifax, Canada - 12 January 1997, Chicago, IL, USA, aged 95.3) Canadian-born American Professor at University of Chicago, Ben May Laboratory for Cancer Research, Chicago, IL, USA, "for his discoveries concerning hormonal treatment of prostatic cancer".

1967 – Granit, Hartline, Wald, Hilleman, Barnard

- The Nobel Prize in Physiology or Medicine 1967 was awarded to **Ragnar Granit**, 67 (30 October 1900, Helsinki, Russian Empire (now Finland) - 12 March 1991, Stockholm, Sweden, aged 90.4), Finnish-born Swedish Professor at Karolinska Institutet, Stockholm, Sweden, **Haldan Keffer Hartline**, 64 (22 December 1903, Bloomsburg, PA, USA - 17 March 1983, Fallston, MD, USA, aged 79.2), American Professor at Rockefeller University, New York, NY, USA, and **George Wald**, 61 (18 November 1906, New York, NY, USA - 12 April 1997, Cambridge, MA, USA, aged 90.4), American Professor at Harvard University, Cambridge, MA, USA, "for their discoveries concerning the primary physiological and chemical visual processes in the eye.

- **Maurice Ralph Hilleman**, 48 (30 August 1919, Miles City, MT – 11 April 2005, Philadelphia, PA, aged 85.6), American microbiologist who specialized in vaccinology, developed the first mumps vaccine – in total he developed a record of over 40 vaccines.

- 3 December - **Christiaan Neethling Barnard**, 45 (8 November 1922, Beaufort West, South Africa – 2 September 2001, Paphos, Cyprus, aged 78.8; he had six children), South African cardiac surgeon who performed the world's first heart transplant, and the first one in which the patient regained consciousness.

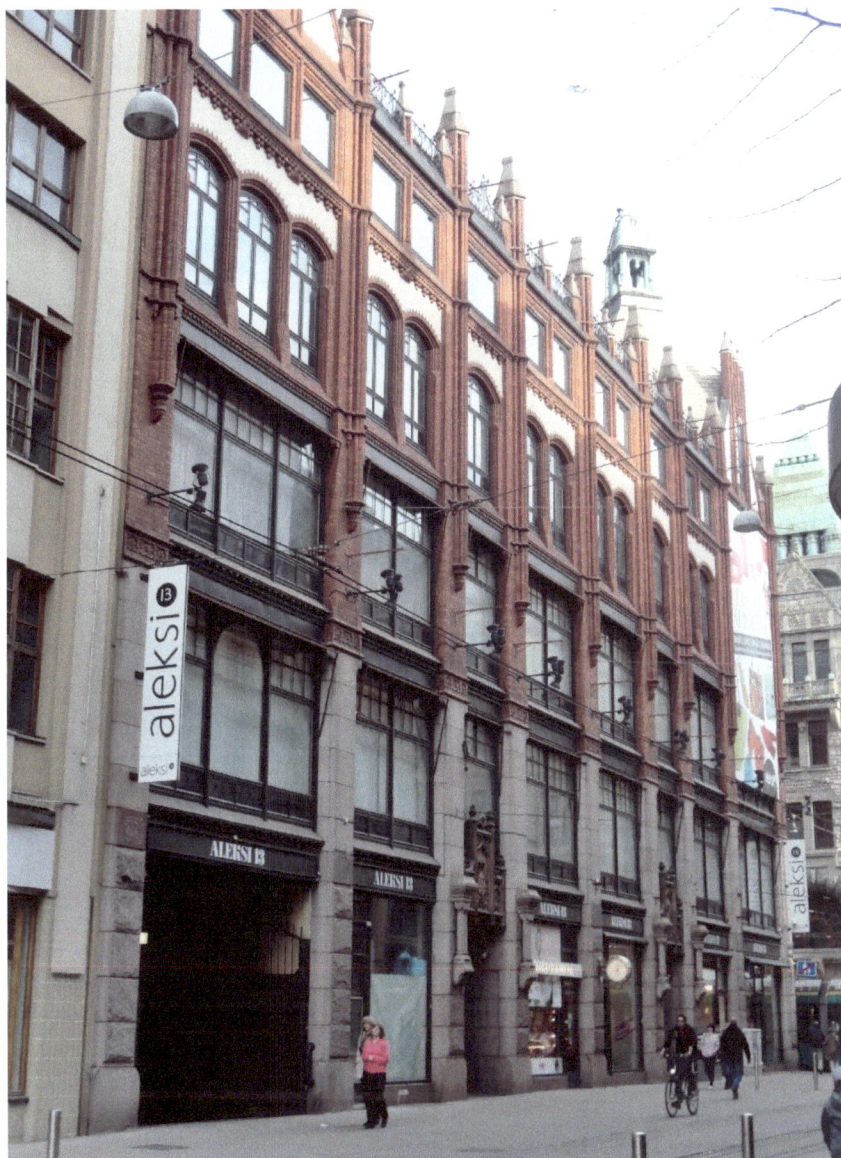

9 May 2013, Finland, Helsinki: beautiful buildings on Mikonkatu, with Aleksi store, close to Aleksanterinkatu, 200 m south-east of the Helsinki Central Railway Station.

1968 – Charcot, Dussik, Holley, Khorana, Nirenberg

- 100 years ago, in 1868, **Jean-Martin Charcot**, 43 (29 November 1825 – 16 August 1893, aged 67.7, French neurologist and professor of anatomical pathology) described and named multiple sclerosis.

- 19 March – Dr. **Karl Dussik**, Austrian psychiatrist, passed away at the age of 60.2 in Lexington, Massachusetts, USA (9 Jan 1908, Vienna, Austria – 19 March 1968, Lexington, Massachusetts, USA). At the hospital in Bad Ischl, Austria, he was the first physician to publish a paper about the medical use of ultrasound: "Further results of the Ultrasonic Investigation of Brain illnesses" presented at the Bad Ischl Ultrasound Symposium, in 1952 (age 44).

- The Nobel Prize in Physiology or Medicine 1968 was awarded to **Robert W. Holley**, 46 (28 January 1922, Urbana, IL, USA - 11 February 1993, Los Gatos, CA, USA, aged 71), American Professor at Cornell University, Ithaca, NY, USA, **Har Gobind Khorana,** 46, (9 January 1922, Raipur, India - 9 November 2011, Concord, MA, USA, aged 89 years and 10 months), Indian-born American Professor at University of Wisconsin, Madison, WI, USA, and **Marshall W. Nirenberg**, 41 (10 April 1927, New York, NY, USA - 15 January 2010, New York, NY, USA, aged 82.6), American Researcher at National Institutes of Health, Bethesda, MD, USA, "for their interpretation of the genetic code and its function in protein synthesis".

1969 – Mendeleev, Cushing, Delbrück, Hershey, Luria

- 6 March – 100 years ago, in 1869, **Dmitri Mendeleev**, 35, (8 February 1834 – 2 February 1907, aged 72.99, 6 days before 73) makes a formal presentation of his periodic table to the Russian Chemical Society. He formulated the Periodic Law, created a wise version of the periodic table of elements, and used it to correct the properties of some already discovered elements, and also to predict the properties of eight elements yet to be discovered.

- 8 April – 100th anniversary of the birth of **Harvey Cushing** (8 April 1869 – 7 October 1939, aged 70.5), American neurosurgeon, pathologist and writer.

- The Nobel Prize in Physiology or Medicine 1969 was awarded to **Max Delbrück**, 63 (4 September 1906, Berlin, Germany - 9 March 1981, Pasadena, CA, USA, aged 74.5), German-born American Professor at California Institute of Technology (Caltech), Pasadena, CA, USA, **Alfred D. Hershey**, 61 (4 December 1908, Owosso, MI, USA - 22 May 1997, Syosset, NY, USA, aged 88.5), American Professor at Carnegie Institution of Washington, Long Island, New York, NY, USA, and **Salvador E. Luria**, 57 (13 August 1912, Torino, Italy - 6 February 1991, Lexington, MA, USA, aged 78.4), Italian-born American Professor at Massachusetts Institute of Technology (MIT), Cambridge, MA, USA, "for their discoveries concerning the replication mechanism and the genetic structure of viruses"

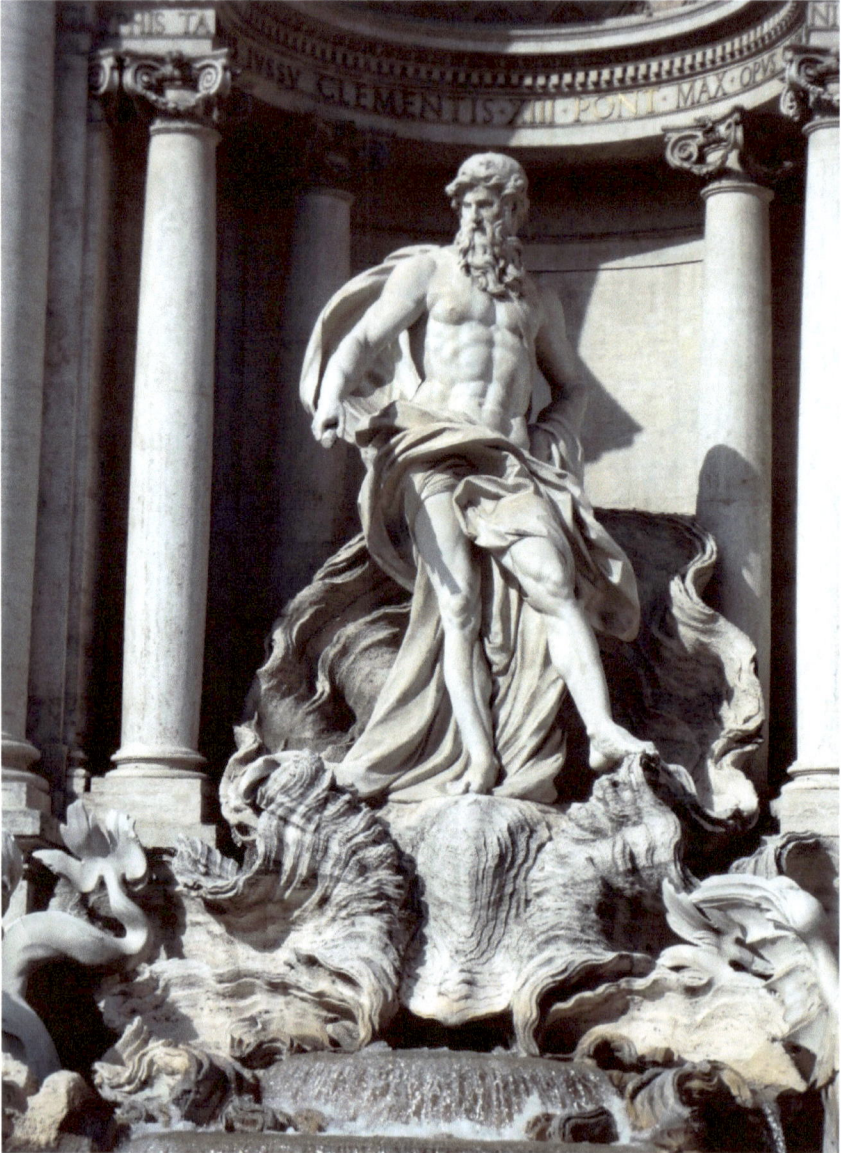

Italy, Roma: Fontana di Trevi (1732 – 1762). Standing 26.3 m high and 49.15 m wide, it is located on Palazzo di Poli (1566). Tritons guide Oceanus' shell chariot, calming hippocampi. In the center an imaginatively modeled triumphal arch is placed over on the palazzo façade. The center niche, or exedra, framing Oceanus, has free-standing columns for greatest light and shade. Pietro Bracci's Oceanus (god of all water) is the central sculpture.

1970 – **Pasteur, Koch, Krogh, Katz, von Euler, Axelrod**

- 100 years ago, in 1870, **Louis Pasteur**, 48, and **Robert Koch**, 27, develop the germs theory of diseases.

- 50 years ago, in 1920, the Nobel Prize in Physiology or Medicine 1920 was awarded to **Schack August Steenberg Krogh**, 46 (15 November 1874, Grenå, Denmark - 13 September 1949, Copenhagen, Denmark, aged 74.8), Danish Professor at Copenhagen University, Copenhagen, Denmark, "for his discovery of the capillary motor regulating mechanism".

- The Nobel Prize in Physiology or Medicine 1970 was awarded to Sir **Bernard Katz**, 59 (26 March 1911, Leipzig, Germany - 20 April 2003, London, United Kingdom, aged 92), German-born British Professor at University College, London, United Kingdom, **Ulf von Euler**, 65 (7 February 1905, Stockholm, Sweden - 9 March 1983, Stockholm, Sweden, aged 78.1; his father Hans von Euler-Chelpin received the Nobel Prize for Chemistry in 1929), Swedish Professor at Karolinska Institutet, Stockholm, Sweden, and **Julius Axelrod**, 58 (30 May 1912, New York, NY, USA - 29 December 2004, Rockville, MD, USA, aged 92.6), American Researcher at National Institutes of Health, Bethesda, MD, USA, "for their discoveries concerning the humoral transmitters in the nerve terminals and the mechanism for their storage, release and inactivation".

- **Maurice Ralph Hilleman**, 51 (30 August 1919, Miles City, MT – 11 April 2005, Philadelphia, PA, aged 85.6), American microbiologist who specialized in vaccinology, developed the first rubella vaccine – in total he developed a record of over 40 vaccines.

1971 – **Galenus, Calmette, Guérin, Sutherland**

- September – 1850th anniversary of the birth of Aelius Galenus or **Claudius Galenus**, or Galen of Pergamum (September 129, Pergamum, Mysia, Anatolia, Roman Empire (now Bergama, Turkey) – 210, Rome, Roman Empire, aged 81), Greek physician, surgeon and philosopher in the Roman Empire. His medical writings influenced the Western and Arab worlds for close to 1500 years, until circa 1700. Galenus rose from gladiators' physician in Asia Minor to court physician in the Rome of Marcus Aurelius (26 April 121, Roma, Roman Empire – 17 March 180, Vindobona, Roman Empire, aged 58.9, called the Philosopher, Roman Emperor for 19 years, from 161 to 180).

- 50 years ago, in 1921, the anti-tuberculosis vaccine was developed after 13 years, from 1908 to 1921, by French bacteriologists **Albert Calmette** and **Camille Guérin**, at the Pasteur Institute in Lille, who named the product Bacillus Calmette-Guérin, or BCG. The vaccine is administered shortly after birth only in infants at high risk of tuberculosis.
Also, in 1921, no Nobel Prize was awarded.

- The Nobel Prize in Physiology or Medicine 1971 was awarded to **Earl W. Sutherland, Jr.,** 56 (19 November 1915, Burlingame, KS, USA - 9 March 1974, Miami, FL, USA, aged 58.3), American Professor at Vanderbilt University, Nashville, TN, USA, "for his discoveries concerning the mechanisms of the action of hormones"

1972 – **Pasteur, Banting, Hill, Meyerhof, Edelman**

- 11 January – 50 years ago, in 1922, insulin was first used in the treatment of diabetes. Insulin was discovered by Sir **Frederick G Banting**, 30, **Charles H Best**, 22, and **JJR Macleod**, 45, at the University of Toronto in 1921, and it was subsequently purified by James B Collip. British professor Ian Murray mentioned that Dr. Nicolae Paulescu (30 Oct 1869 – 17 July 1931, aged 61.7) independently discovered insulin (which he called pancreine) 5 years before, in 1916 (age 47), and he secured the patent rights for his method of manufacturing pancreine on 10 April 1922. In 1910, Sir Edward Albert Sharpey-Shafer suggested only one chemical was missing from the pancreas in people with diabetes. He called this chemical insulin, which comes for the Latin word insula, meaning "island".

- 11 August - **Max Theiler,** South African-American virologist and physician, passed away at the age of 73.6 (30 Jan 1899, Pretoria South Africa – 11 August 1972, New Haven, CT, USA). He was awarded the Nobel Prize in Physiology or Medicine in 1951, age 52, for developing a vaccine against yellow fever in 1937, at age 38.

- October - the First International Conference on Computer Communications is held in Washington, D.C., and hosts the first public demonstration of ARPAnet, a precursor of the Internet.

- 27 December – 150th anniversary of the birth of **Louis Pasteur** (27 December 1822, Dole, France – 28 September 1895, Marnes-la-Coquette, France, aged 72.7), French biologist, microbiologist and chemist, renowned for his discoveries of the principles of vaccination, microbial fermentation, and pasteurization. He is remembered for his remarkable breakthroughs in the causes and prevention of diseases, and his discoveries have saved many lives ever since. Quotes:
In the fields of observation chance favors only the prepared mind.

Science knows no country, because knowledge belongs to humanity, and is the torch which illuminates the world.

There are no such things as applied sciences, only applications of science.

- 50 years ago, in 1922, the Nobel Prize in Physiology or Medicine 1922 was awarded to **Archibald Vivian Hill**, 36 (26 September 1886, Bristol, United Kingdom - 3 June 1977, Cambridge, United Kingdom, aged 90 years 9 months and 23 days), British Professor at London University, London, United Kingdom, "for his discovery, during the 1910s, relating to the production of heat in the muscle", and **Otto Fritz Meyerhof**, 38 (12 April 1884, Hanover, Germany - 6 October 1951, Philadelphia, PA, USA, after two heart attacks in 1944 and 1951, aged 67.5), German Professor at Kiel University, Kiel, Germany, "for his discovery, at the end of the 1910s, of the fixed relationship between the consumption of oxygen and the metabolism of lactic acid in the muscle".

- The Nobel Prize in Physiology or Medicine 1972 was awarded to **Gerald M. Edelman**, 43 (1 July 1929, New York, NY, USA - 17 May 2014, La Jolla, CA, USA, aged 84.9), American Professor at Rockefeller University, New York, NY, USA, and **Rodney R. Porter**, 55 (8 October 1917, Newton-le-Willows, United Kingdom - 6 September 1985, Winchester, United Kingdom, aged 67.9), British Professor at University of Oxford, Oxford, United Kingdom, "for their discoveries concerning the chemical structure of antibodies".

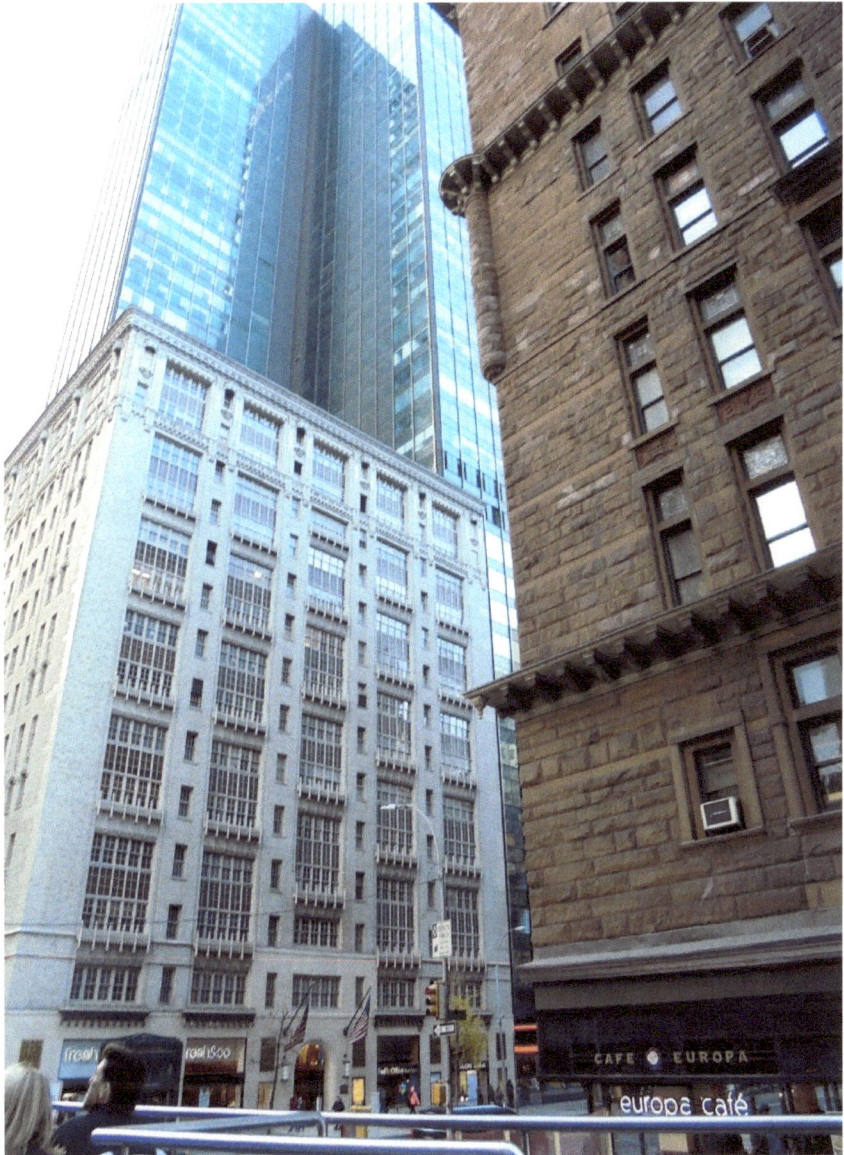

On 7th Avenue at West 57th Street, looking southwest: right: a classical building, which is tangent to the right, on W 57th St, to the American Fine Arts Society building (1892); left down: a beautiful building, opposite Carnegie Hall (to the left, across 7th Ave, 1891, concert hall with exceptional acoustics, architecture and performance history); left up: an impressive double skyscraper, with the southwest side on W 56th St.

Chapter 4. 1973 – 1982: Avicenna, Harvey, della Torre, Wren, van Leeuwenhoek, Laennec, Davy

1973 – van Leeuwenhoek, White, Macleod, von Frisch

- 300 years ago, in 1673, **Antonie van Leeuwenhoek**, 41, (24 Oct 1632 – 26 August 1723, aged 90.8, Dutch microbiologist) was the first to observe microbes with a homemade microscope.

- 31 October - **Paul Dudley White**, American physician and cardiologist, passed away at the age of 87.3 in Boston, Massachusetts, USA (6 June 1886, Roxbury, Boston, MA, USA – 31 Oct 1973, Boston, Massachusetts, USA). He graduated Harvard College and Harvard Medical School, was one of the leading cardiologists of his day, a founding member of the American Heart Association, and a prominent advocate of preventive medicine. In 1913, Dr. Paul Dudley White, 27, pioneered the use of the electrocardiograph – ECG.

- 50 years ago, in 1923, **Frederick Banting**, 32 (14 November 1891, Alliston, Canada - 21 February 1941, killed in an air disaster in Newfoundland, Canada, aged 49.3), Canadian Professor at University of Toronto, Toronto, Canada, and **John James Rickard Macleod**, 47 (6 September 1876, Cluny, Scotland - 16 March 1935, Aberdeen, Scotland, aged 58.5), British Professor at University of Toronto, Toronto, Canada, received the Nobel Prize in Physiology or Medicine 1923, for discovering insulin in 1921 - Frederick Banting suspected that another substance formed in the pancreas, trypsin, broke down the insulin. In John MacLeod's laboratory, on 14 April 1921, Frederick Banting and Charles Best treated dogs so that they no longer produced trypsin. Insulin could then be extracted and used to treat diabetes. Banting mentioned in his Nobel Lecture "Diabetes and Insulin", on 15 September 1925, that "The problem of the extraction of the antidiabetic principle from the pancreas was then taken up for the most part by physiologists among whom were Scott, Paulesco, Kleiner, and Murlin." Macleod mentioned in his Nobel Lecture "The Physiology of Insulin and Its Source in the Animal Body", on 26 May 1925, that "Special reference must also be made to the more recent work of Paulesco who prepared extracts having very decided effects on the sugar and the urea of the blood of diabetic animals."

- The Nobel Prize in Physiology or Medicine 1973 was awarded to **Karl von Frisch**, 87 (20 November 1886, Vienna, Austria - 12 June 1982, Munich, West Germany (now Germany), aged 95.6), Austrian-born German Professor at Zoologisches Institut der Universität München, Munich, Federal Republic of Germany, **Konrad Lorenz**, 70 (7 November 1903, Vienna, Austria - 27 February 1989, Vienna, Austria, aged 85.3), Austrian Professor at Konrad-Lorenz-Institut der Österreichischen Akademie der Wissenschaften, Forschungsstelle für Ethologie, Altenberg; Grünau im Almtal, Austria, and **Nikolaas Tinbergen**, 66 (15 April 1907, the Hague, the Netherlands - 21 December 1988, Oxford, United Kingdom, aged 81.6), Dutch-born British Professor at University of Oxford, Oxford, United Kingdom, "for their discoveries concerning organization and elicitation of individual and social behavior patterns".

1974 – Einthoven, Claude, de Duve, Palade, Takahashi

- April - the world population reaches 4 billions of people, estimated by the United States Census Bureau.

- 50 years ago, in 1924, the Nobel Prize in Physiology or Medicine 1924 was awarded to **Willem Einthoven**, 64 (21 May 1860, Semarang, Java, Dutch East Indies (now Indonesia) - 29 September 1927, Leiden, the Netherlands, aged 67.3), Dutch Professor at Leiden University, Leiden, the Netherlands, for his discovery of the mechanism of the electrocardiogram (ECG) - Willem Einthoven developed doctors' ability to depict the heart and its parts, functions, and illnesses using ECGs. One key to this progress (and to avoid complex mathematical corrections), was the string galvanometer, which precisely measures tiny currents, constructed by Willem Einthoven in 1903, at age 43.

- The Nobel Prize in Physiology or Medicine 1974 was awarded to **Albert Claude**, 76 (24 August 1898, Longlier, Belgium - 22 May 1983, Brussels, Belgium, aged 84.7), Belgian Professor at Université Catholique de Louvain, Louvain, Belgium, **Christian de Duve**, 57 (2 October 1917, Thames Ditton, United Kingdom - 4 May 2013, Nethen, Belgium, aged 95.6), British-born American Professor at Rockefeller University, New York, NY, USA, Université Catholique de Louvain, Louvain, Belgium, and **George E. Palade**, 62 (19 November 1912, Iasi, Romania - 7 October 2008, Del Mar, CA, USA, aged 95.9, just 43 days before 96), Romanian-born American Professor at Yale University, School of Medicine, New Haven, CT, USA, "for their discoveries concerning the structural and functional organization of the cell".

- **Michiaki Takahashi**, 46 (17 February 1928, Osaka, Japan — 16 December 2013, Osaka, aged 85.8), Japanese physician and virologist, developed the first vaccine for chickenpox.

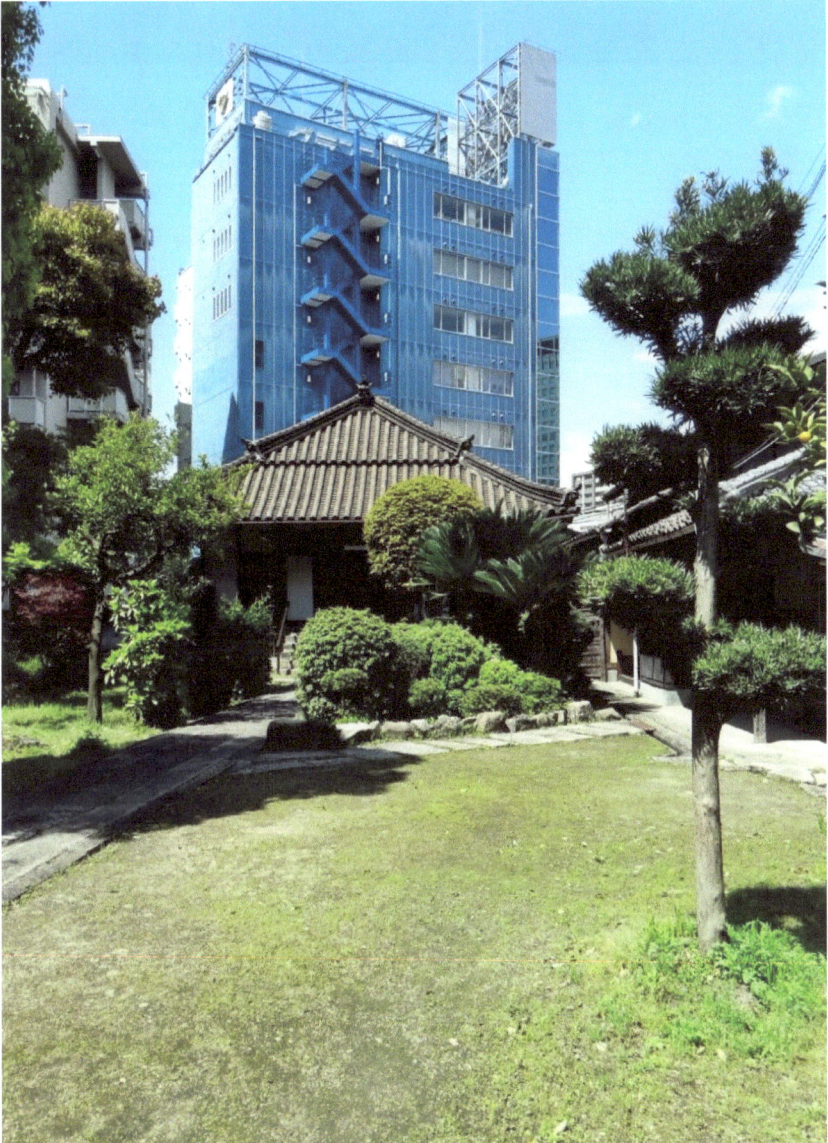

Japan, Osaka (which means "large hill" or "large slope", in 645 capital, 400 km west of Tokyo, the second largest city after Tokyo, metropolitan area around has 19,000,000 people, along with Paris and London is one of the most productive city in the world with a GDP of $341 billion, situated at the mouth of the Yodo River on Osaka Bay of the Pacific Ocean), a small Buddhist Temple west of Shin Osaka Washington Plaza Hotel and southwest of Shin Osaka Station (1964, 2011, 3 km from the older Osaka Station).

1975 – Avicenna, Landois, Baltimore, Dulbecco, Ledley

- 950 years ago, in 1025, the Canon of Medicine by **Avicenna** (22 August 980, in Samanid Empire (now Uzbekistan) – 21 June 1037, in Kakuyid Emirate (now Iran), aged 56.8, Persian polymath who is regarded as one of the most significant physicians, astronomers, thinkers and writers of that period) set the standard medical textbook for over 700 years, through 18th century, in Europe. After 948 years, in 1973, Avicenna's Canon of Medicine was reprinted in New York.

- 100 years ago, in 1875, **Leonard Landois**, 38 (1 December 1837 – 17 November 1902, aged 64.9, German physiologist) had reported that, when to a man it is given transfusions of the blood of other animals, these foreign blood corpuscles are clumped and broken up in the blood vessels of the man, with the liberation of haemoglobin.

- 50 years ago, in 1925, no Nobel Prize was awarded.

- The Nobel Prize in Physiology or Medicine 1975 was awarded to **David Baltimore**, 37 (born: 7 March 1938, New York, NY, USA), American Professor at Massachusetts Institute of Technology (MIT), Cambridge, MA, USA, **Renato Dulbecco**, 59 (22 February 1914, Catanzaro, Italy - 19 February 2012, La Jolla, CA, USA, aged 97.99, just 3 days before 98), Italian-born British Researcher at Imperial Cancer Research Fund Laboratory, London, United Kingdom), and **Howard Martin Temin**, 41 (10 December 1934, Philadelphia, PA, USA - 9 February 1994, Madison, WI, USA, aged 59.2), American Professor at University of Wisconsin, Madison, WI, USA, "for their discoveries concerning the interaction between tumor viruses and the genetic material of the cell".

- **Robert Steven Ledley**, 49 (28 June 1926, New York City – 24 July 2012, Kensington, MD, aged 86), American Professor of Physiology and Biophysics and Professor of Radiology at Georgetown University School of Medicine, also mathematician, invented the full-body Computer Tomography (CT) scanner.

1976 – Bojanus, Fibiger, Blumberg, Gajdusek

- 16 July – 200th anniversary of the birth of **Ludwig Heinrich Bojanus** (July 16, 1776 – April 2, 1827, aged 50.7), German physician and naturalist, professor at Vilnius University in Russia. In 1814 he was elected corresponding member of the Imperial Academy of Sciences in St. Petersburg; in 1818 he became a member of the Imperial Leopold-Caroline Academy of Natural Sciences in Bonn, and in 1821 was a foreign member of the Royal Swedish Academy of Sciences.

- January - the Cray-1, the first commercially developed supercomputer, is released by Seymour Cray's (1925 – 1996, aged 71) mathematician and electrical engineer) Cray Research.

- 50 years ago, in 1926, the Nobel Prize in Physiology or Medicine 1926 was awarded to **Johannes Andreas Grib Fibiger**, 59 (23 April 1867, Silkeborg, Denmark - 30 January 1928, Copenhagen, Denmark, of cardiac failure with multiple emboli and massive pulmonary infarcts, also cancer of the colon: caecostomy, aged 60.7), Danish Professor at Copenhagen University, Copenhagen, Denmark, "for his discovery of the Spiroptera carcinoma".

- The Nobel Prize in Physiology or Medicine 1976 was awarded to **Baruch S. Blumberg**, 51 (28 July 1925, New York, NY, USA - 5 April 2011, Moffett Field, CA, USA, aged 85.7), American Researcher at The Institute for Cancer Research, Philadelphia, PA, USA, and **D. Carleton Gajdusek**, 53 (9 September 1923, Yonkers, NY, USA - 12 December 2008, Tromsø, Norway, aged 85.2), American Researcher at National Institutes of Health, Bethesda, MD, USA, "for their discoveries concerning new mechanisms for the origin and dissemination of infectious diseases".

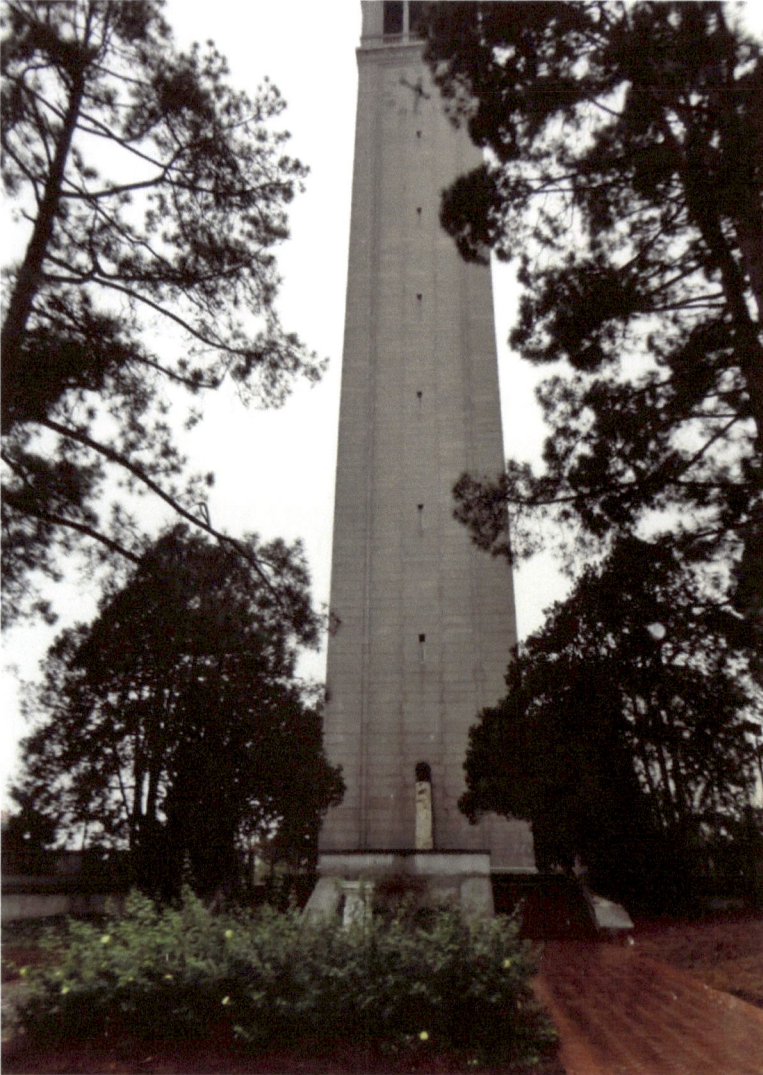

USA, the University of California, Berkeley (1868, named after the philosopher and mathematician Bishop George Berkeley (1685-1753), motto Fiat lux (Let there be light), 36,200 students, major public research university, 72 Nobel laureates, between the top six universities in the world, 500 ha campus), il Campanile (Sather Tower (61 bells (full concert carillon) and clock tower). 1914, 94 m, 7 floors, observation deck on the 8th floor, inspired by il Campanile (850, 1514, 1912, 99 m) di San Marco (1084), Venezia (421, Venice), Italy (900 BC)).

1977 – Lister, Wagner-Jauregg, Guillemin, Austrian

- 5 April – 150th anniversary of the birth of **Joseph Lister** (5 April 1827, Upton House, Newham, UK – 10 Feb 1912, Walmer, UK, aged 84.8), British surgeon and a pioneer of antiseptic surgery. He promoted, in 1867 (age 40), the idea of sterile surgery while working at the Glasgow Royal Infirmary, and published Antiseptic Principle of the Practice of Surgery.

- 50 years ago, in 1927, the Nobel Prize in Physiology or Medicine 1927 was awarded to **Julius Wagner-Jauregg**, 70 (7 March 1857, Wels, Austria - 27 September 1940, Vienna, Austria, aged 83.5), Austrian Professor at Vienna University, Vienna, Austria, "for his discovery of the therapeutic value of malaria inoculation in the treatment of dementia paralytica - in 1917, Julius Wagner-Jauregg, 60, exposed patients with mental illnesses and general paralysis to malaria-infected blood, and could in this way cure or alleviate general paralysis. The malaria was of a type that was comparatively innocuous, and consequently the patient's health could be improved.

- The Nobel Prize in Physiology or Medicine 1977 was awarded to Roger Guillemin, 53 (born: 11 January 1924, Dijon, France), French-born American Researcher at The Salk Institute, San Diego, CA, USA, and Andrew V. Schally, 51 (born: 30 November 1926, Wilno (now Vilnius), Poland (now Lithuania)), Polish-born American Researcher at Veterans Administration Hospital, New Orleans, LA, USA, "for their discoveries concerning the peptide hormone production of the brain", and Rosalyn Yalow, 56 (19 July 1921, New York, NY, USA - 30 May 2011, New York, NY, USA, aged 89.9), American Researcher at Veterans Administration Hospital, Bronx, NY, USA, "for the development of radioimmunoassays of peptide hormones".

- **Robert Austrian**, 61 (12 April 1916, Baltimore – 25 March 2007, Philadelphia, aged 90 years 11 months and 13 days),

American infectious diseases physician, developed the first pneumococcal vaccine against the Streptococcus pneumoniae.

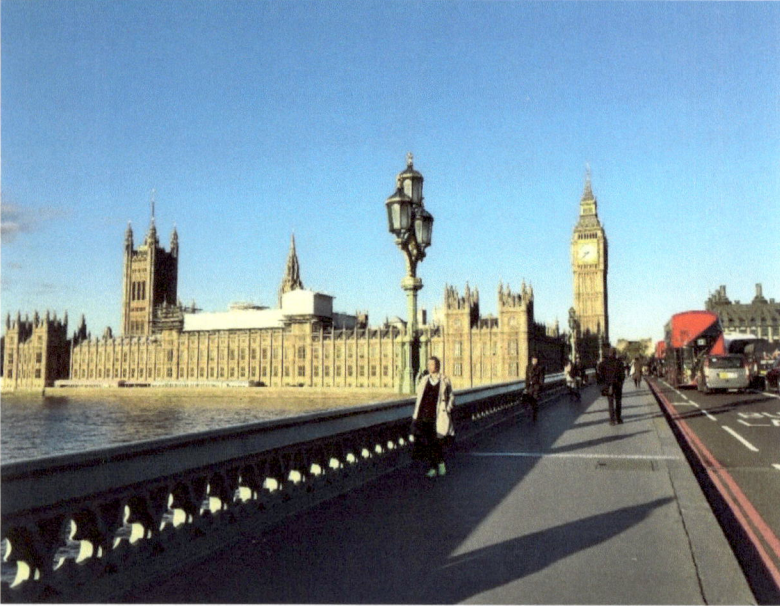

From the Westminster Bridge (1862, 250 m) over Thames (flowing left to right), looking west to the Palace of Westminster (1016, 1870, left), Big Ben (Elizabeth Tower, 1855, 96 m, center right), and to Portcullis House (2001, right).

1978 – Harvey, Davy, Nicolle, Edwards, Arber, Nathans

- 1 April – 400th anniversary of the birth of **William Harvey** (1 April 1578, Folkestone, United Kingdom – 3 June 1657, Roehampton, London, United Kingdom, aged 79.1), English physician who made important contributions in anatomy and physiology. In 1628 (age 50) he published in Latin at Frankfurt his completed treatise on the circulation of the blood, the De Motu Cordis. Quotes:

All we know is still infinitely less than all that remains unknown.

I profess both to learn and to teach anatomy, not from books but from dissections; not from positions of philosophers but from the fabric of nature.

I avow myself the partisan of truth alone.

There is a lust in man no charm can tame:
Of loudly publishing his neighbor's shame:
On eagles wings immortal scandals fly,
While virtuous actions are born and die.

- 17 December - 200th anniversary of the birth of Sir **Humphry Davy** (17 Dec 1778, Penzance, UK – 29 May 1829, Geneva, Switzerland, aged 50.4), Cornish chemist and inventor, who is best remembered today for isolating, using electricity, a series of elements for the first time: potassium, sodium, magnesium, calcium, strontium, boron, chlorine, iodine, and barium. In 1800 Sir Humphry Davy, 22, discovered the anesthetics properties of nitrous oxide.

- 28 September - 50 years ago, in 1928 - discovery of penicillin by Sir **Alexander Fleming**, 47. He gave the name penicillin on 7 March 1929. He received the Nobel Prize in 1945.

Also, in 1928, the Nobel Prize in Physiology or Medicine 1928 was awarded to **Charles Jules Henri Nicolle**, 62 (21 September 1866, Rouen, France - 28 February 1936, Tunis, Tunisia, aged 69.6), French Director of the Pasteur Institute in Tunis, for his work on typhus - in 1909, at the age of 43, he demonstrated that body lice spread typhus.

- 25 July - the first child was born as a result of in vitro fertilization, which was developed by **Robert G. Edwards**, 53, (27 Sep 1925, Batley, UK – 10 April 2013, Cambridge, UK, aged 87.6), British Professor at University of Cambridge, Cambridge, United Kingdom. He received the Nobel Prize in Physiology or Medicine in 2010 (age 85) "for the development of in vitro fertilization".

- The Nobel Prize in Physiology or Medicine 1978 was awarded to **Werner Arber**, 49 (born: 3 June 1929, Gränichen, Switzerland), Swiss Professor at Biozentrum der Universität, Basel, Switzerland, **Daniel Nathans**, 50 (30 October 1928, Wilmington, DE, USA - 16 November 1999, Baltimore, MD, USA, aged 71), American Professor at Johns Hopkins University School of Medicine, Baltimore, MD, USA, and **Hamilton O. Smith**, 47 (born: 23 August 1931, New York, NY, USA), American Professor at Johns Hopkins University School of Medicine, Baltimore, MD, USA, "for the discovery of restriction enzymes and their application to problems of molecular genetics".

- The first vaccine for meningitis (Neisseria meningitidis) -- meningococcal polysaccharide vaccine or MPSV4 -- was developed by Sanofi Pasteur.

1979 – Huygens, Forssmann, Eijkman, Hopkins, Cormack

14 April – 350th anniversary of the birth of **Christaan Huygens** (14 April 1629 – 8 July 1695, aged 66.2, founder of mathematical physics, contributions in optics and mechanics, discovered Saturn's moon Titan, invention of the Huygenian eyepiece for the telescope, and invented the pendulum clock in 1656, which was a breakthrough in timekeeping, and became the most accurate timekeeper for almost 300 years)

- 100 years ago, in 1879, **Louis Pasteur**, 57, discovered the first vaccine, with a disease called chicken cholera. After accidentally exposing chickens to the attenuated form of a culture, he demonstrated that they became resistant to the actual virus.

- 50 years ago, in 1929, **Werner Forssmann**, 25, succeeded in inserting a catheter into his own heart. From the crook of his arm he inserted a thin catheter through a vein into his heart and took an X-ray photo. He inserted a cannula into his own antecubital vein, through which he passed a catheter for 65 cm, and then walked to the X-ray department, where a photograph was taken of the catheter lying in his right auricle. The experiment paved the way for many types of heart studies.
- Also in 1929, the Nobel Prize in Physiology or Medicine 1929 was awarded to **Christiaan Eijkman**, 71 (11 August 1858, Nijkerk, the Netherlands - 5 November 1930, Utrecht, the Netherlands, aged 72.2), Dutch Professor at Utrecht University, Utrecht, the Netherlands, for his discovery of the antineuritic vitamin - in 1897, age 39, he concluded that there was a substance in the husk of rice that counteracted the beriberi (which was associated with the consumption of decorticated rice); these vital substances came to be called vitamins; the substance that counteracts beriberi subsequently was designated vitamin B1, and Sir **Frederick Gowland Hopkins**, 68 (20 June 1861, Eastbourne, United Kingdom - 16 May 1947, Cambridge, United Kingdom, aged 85.9), British Professor at University of Cambridge, Cambridge, United Kingdom, for his discovery of the growth-stimulating vitamins – he reported around 1910 that there are some unknown

substances that are necessary in small amounts for life processes. The substances came to be known as vitamins.

- The Nobel Prize in Physiology or Medicine 1979 was awarded to **Allan M. Cormack**, 55 (23 February 1924, Johannesburg, South Africa - 7 May 1998, Winchester, MA, USA, aged 74.2), South African-born American Professor at Tufts University, Medford, MA, USA, and **Godfrey N. Hounsfield**, 60 (28 August 1919, Newark, United Kingdom - 12 August 2004, Kingston upon Thames, United Kingdom, aged 84.9), British Researcher at Central Research Laboratories, EMI, London, United Kingdom, "for the development of computer assisted tomography".

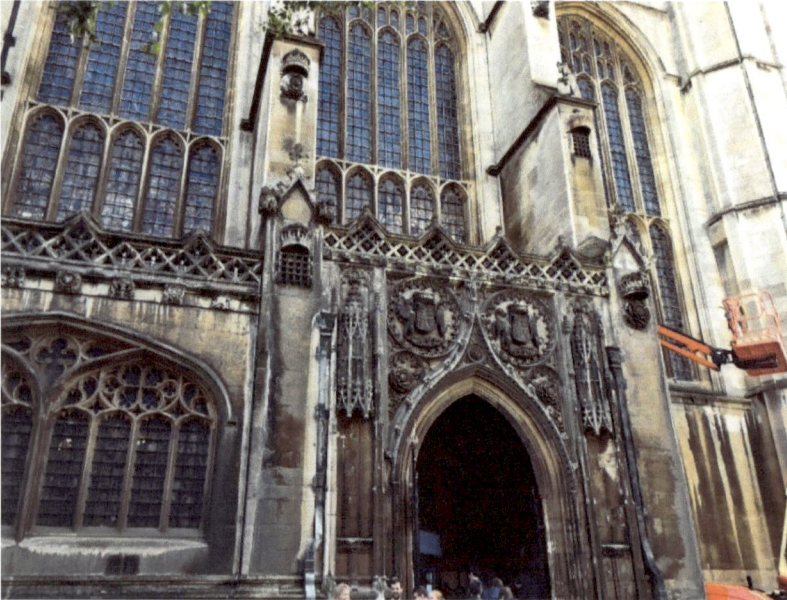

Cambridge, UK: From Trinity Lane looking south to the west part of the northern façade and entrance of King's College Chapel (1446).

1980 – Landsteiner, Reichstein, Benacerraf, Dausset, Snell

- 22 August – 1000th anniversary of the birth of **Avicenna** (22 August 980, in Samanid Empire (now Uzbekistan) – 21 June 1037, in Kakuyid Emirate (now Iran), aged 56.8), Persian polymath, who is regarded as one of the most significant physicians, astronomers, thinkers and writers of that period. In 1010 Avicenna, 30, wrote The Book of Healing, and in 1025, at the age of 45, he wrote The Canon of Medicine, which set the standard medical textbook for over 700 years, through 18th century, in Europe. After 948 years, in 1973, Avicenna's Canon of Medicine was reprinted in New York.

- 50 years ago, in 1930, **Karl Landsteiner**, 62 (14 June 1868, Vienna, Austrian Empire (now Austria) - 26 June 1943, New York, NY, USA, of heart attack in his laboratory, aged 75 years and 12 days), Austrian-born American Professor at Rockefeller Institute for Medical Research, New York, NY, USA, was awarded the Nobel Prize in Physiology or Medicine 1930 for his description of the human ABO blood group system in 1901, at age 33.

Also, in 1930, **Tadeus Reichstein**, 33, who received the Nobel Prize in Physiology or Medicine 1950, found that the aroma of coffee is composed of extremely complex substances, among which are derivatives of furan and pyrrole, and substances containing sulphur.

- The Nobel Prize in Physiology or Medicine 1980 was awarded to **Baruj Benacerraf**, 60 (29 October 1920, Caracas, Venezuela - 2 August 2011, Boston, MA, USA, aged 90.7), Venezuelan-born American Professor at Harvard Medical School, Boston, MA, USA, **Jean Dausset**, 64 (19 October 1916, Toulouse, France - 6 June 2009, Palma, Majorca, Spain, aged 92.6), French Professor at Université de Paris, Laboratoire Immuno-Hématologie, Paris, France, and **George D. Snell**, 77 (19 December 1903, Bradford, MA, USA - 6 June 1996, Bar Harbor, ME, USA, aged 92.5), American Researcher at Jackson Laboratory, Bar Harbor, ME, USA, "for their discoveries concerning genetically determined structures on the cell surface that regulate immunological reactions".

- Smallpox was declared eradicated worldwide, due to vaccination efforts.

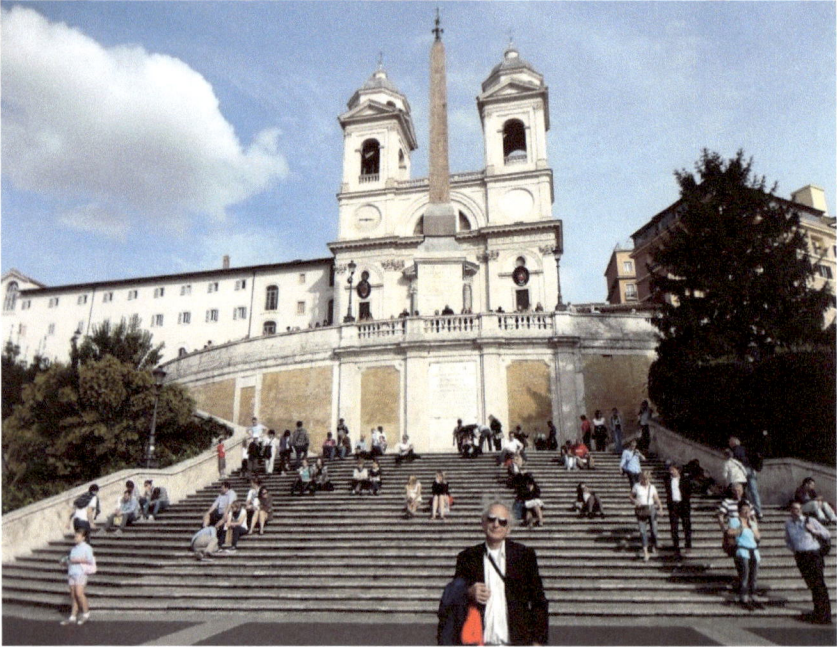

Italy, Roma: Trinità dei Monti church, 1585, with Obelisco Sallustiano (20 BC), and Scalinata della Trinità dei Monti (the Spanish Steps, 1725).

1981 – della Torre, Laennec, Warburg, Sperry, Murray,

- 500th anniversary of the birth of **Marcantonio della Torre** (1481, Verona, Italy – 1511, Riva del Garda, Italy, aged 30), Italian precocious child, who received the doctorate in philosophy on 22 December 1497, at age 16, and in medicine on 1 February 1501, at age 20, at the University of Padua, then was Professor of Anatomy, who lectured at the University of Pavia and at the University of Padua. He collaborated with Leonardo da Vinci for his Anatomy books, in the last two years of his very short life – 1510 and 1511.

- 17 February - 200th anniversary of the birth of **René-Théophile-Hyacinthe Laennec** (17 Feb 1781, Quimper, Brittany, France -13 August 1826 of tuberculosis, Ploaré, France, aged 45.5), French physician, who invented the stethoscope in 1816 (age 35, when he was unable to feel a patient's heartbeat through his hand or by pressing his ear, especially on women's chests (he was very shy)), while working at the Hôpital Necker, and pioneered its use in diagnosing various chest conditions. He became a lecturer at the Collège de France in 1822 (age 41) and professor of medicine in 1823, at age 42, for less than 3 years.

- 100 years ago, in 1881, **Louis Pasteur**, 59, developed the first vaccine for anthrax, which was used successfully in sheep, goats and cows.

50 years ago, in 1931, the Nobel Prize in Physiology or Medicine 1931 was awarded to **Otto Heinrich Warburg**, 48 (8 October 1883, Freiburg im Breisgau, Germany - 1 August 1970, West Berlin, West Germany (now Germany), aged 86.9), German Professor at Kaiser-Wilhelm-Institut (now Max-Planck-Institut) für Biologie, Berlin-Dahlem, Germany, for his discovery of the nature and mode of action of the respiratory enzyme - in 1928, age 45, he concluded that the respiration enzyme, he was looking for, was a red ferrous pigment related to the blood pigment, hemoglobin.

- 12 August - the IBM Personal Computer is released.

- The Nobel Prize in Physiology or Medicine 1981 was awarded to **Roger W. Sperry**, 68 (20 August 1913, Hartford, CT, USA - 17 April 1994, Pasadena, CA, USA, aged 80.6), American Professor at California Institute of Technology (Caltech), Pasadena, CA, USA, "for his discoveries concerning the functional specialization of the cerebral hemispheres", **David H. Hubel**, 55 (27 February 1926, Windsor, ON, Canada - 22 September 2013, Lincoln, MA, USA, aged 87.6), Canadian-born American Professor at Harvard Medical School, Boston, MA, USA, and **Torsten N. Wiesel**, 57 (born: 3 June 1924, Uppsala, Sweden), Swedish-born American Professor at Harvard Medical School, Boston, MA, USA, "for their discoveries concerning information processing in the visual system".

- Sir **Kenneth Murray**, 51 (30 December 1930, East Ardsley, West Riding of Yorkshire, England — 7 April 2013, Edinburgh, UK, aged 82.3), British molecular biologist, developed the vaccine against hepatitis B, and he is one of the founders of Biogen.

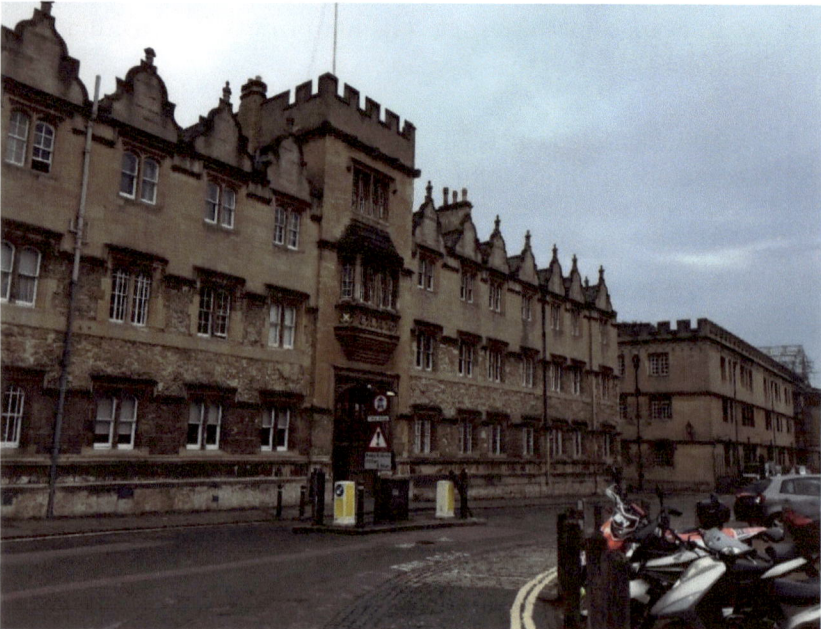

Oxford, UK: On Oriel Street, looking to the west façade of Oriel College (1326), Merton St, Corpus Christy College (1517, right).

1982 – Wren, Sherrington, Adrian, Bergström, Samuelsson

- 24 October - 350th anniversary of the birth of **Antonie Philips van Leeuwenhoek** (24 Oct 1632, Delft, Netherlands, - 26 August 1723, Delft, Netherlands, aged 90.8, FRS), Dutch businessman and scientist in the Golden Age of Dutch science and technology. A largely self-taught man in science, he is known as "the Father of Microbiology", and one of the first microscopists and microbiologists. In 1670, Antonie van Leeuwenhoek, 38, discovered blood cells, and in 1683, at age 51, he observed bacteria. Microbiology started with Antonie van Leeuwenhoek in 1676, when he was 44.

- 30 October – 350th anniversary of the birth of Sir **Christopher Wren** (30 Oct 1632, East Knoyle, United Kingdom – 8 March 1723, St James's, London, United Kingdom, aged 90.3, buried on 16 March 1723, in St. Paul's Cathedral, City of London, United Kingdom), English mathematician, anatomist, astronomer, physicist, and one of the most highly acclaimed English architects in history. In 1656, Sir Christopher Wren, 24, experimented with canine blood transfusions. It is interesting that Wren was 6 days younger than van Leeuwenhoek, and died at the age of 90 years 4 months and 8 days, 5 months and 18 days before van Leeuwenhoek, who died at the age of 90 years 10 months and 2 days.

- 100 years ago, in 1882, **Louis Pasteur**, 60, developed the first vaccine against rabies.

- 100 years ago, in 1882, **Robert Koch**, 39, was the first microbiologist to report the successful isolation of the causative agent of tuberculosis, named 1 year later as Mycobacterium tuberculosis.

50 years ago, in 1932, the Nobel Prize in Physiology or Medicine 1932 was awarded to, Sir **Charles Scott Sherrington**, 75 (27 November 1857, London, United Kingdom - 4 March 1952, Eastbourne, United Kingdom, of heart failure, aged 94 years 3 months and 5 days), British Professor at University of Oxford,

Oxford, United Kingdom, and **Edgar Douglas Adrian**, 43 (30 November 1889, London, United Kingdom - 8 August 1977, Cambridge, United Kingdom, aged 87.6), British Professor at University of Cambridge, Cambridge, United Kingdom, for their discoveries regarding the functions of neurons - in the 1890s Charles Sherrington showed how muscular contractions are followed by relaxation, and how different reflexes are part of a complicated interplay, in which the spinal cord and brain process nerve impulses, and turn them into new impulses to muscles and organs. In 1886 Sherrington, 31, stayed with Koch, 43, to do research in bacteriology for a year. During the First World War, as Chairman of the Industrial Fatigue Board, he worked for a time in a shell factory at Birmingham, and the daily shift of 13 hours, with a Sunday shift of 9 hours, did not, at the age of 57, tire him. Edgar Adrian developed methods for measuring electrical signals in the nervous system, and in 1928, age 39, he found that these always have a certain size. More intensive stimuli do not result in stronger signals, but rather signals that are sent more often and through more nerve fibers.

- The Nobel Prize in Physiology or Medicine 1982 was awarded to **Sune K. Bergström**, 66 (10 January 1916, Stockholm, Sweden - 15 August 2004, Stockholm, Sweden, aged 88.7), Swedish Professor at Karolinska Institutet, Stockholm, Sweden, **Bengt I. Samuelsson**, 48 (born: 21 May 1934, Halmstad, Sweden), Swedish Professor at Karolinska Institutet, Stockholm, Sweden, and **John R. Vane**,55 (29 March 1927, Tardebigg, United Kingdom - 19 November 2004, Farnborough, United Kingdom, aged 77.6), British Researcher at The Wellcome Research Laboratories, Beckenham, United Kingdom, "for their discoveries concerning prostaglandins and related biologically active substances".

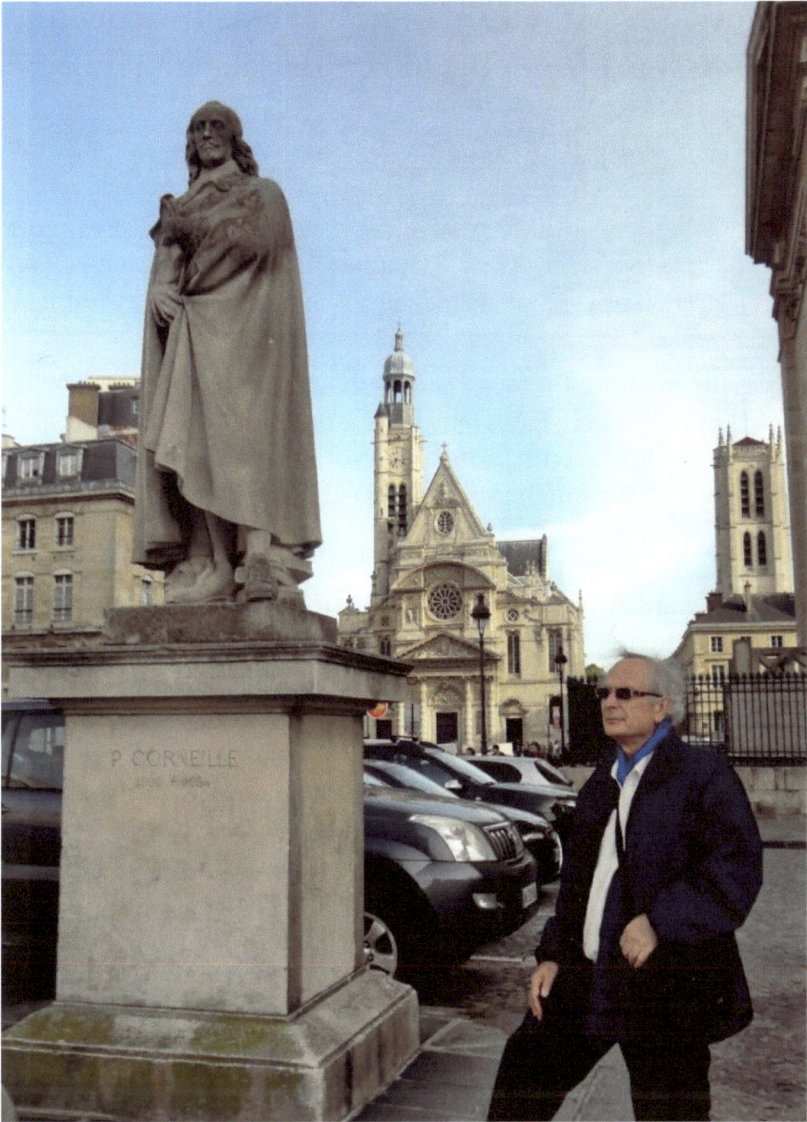

The statue of Pierre Corneille (1606 – 1684, poet and dramatist, the creator of French classical tragedy (Le Cid, Horace, Cinna, La Place royale), one of the three great 17th century French dramatists, along with Molière (1622 – 1673) and Racine (1639 – 1699)) and Paroisse Saint-Étienne-du-Mont (center, 510, 1222, 1328, 1492-1626) – a Catholic church, north-east of the Panthéon (right), with the tombs of Blaise Pascal (1623 – 1662, mathematician, physicist, philosopher, inventor and writer) and Jean-Baptiste Racine.

Chapter 5. 1983 – 1992: Hippocrates, Dioscorides, Janssen, Blundell, Fahrenheit, Lavoisier

1983 – Magendie, Reichstein, Morgan

- 6 October - 200th anniversary of the birth of **François Magendie** (6 October 1783 – 7 October 1855, aged 72 years and one day), French physiologist, pioneer of experimental physiology.

- 50 years ago, in 1933, **Tadeus Reichstein**, 36, who received the Nobel Prize in Physiology or Medicine 1950, succeeded, independently of Sir Norman Haworth and his collaborators in Birmingham, in synthesizing vitamin C (ascorbic acid).

Also in 1933, the Nobel Prize in Physiology or Medicine 1933 was awarded to **Thomas Hunt Morgan**, 67 (25 September 1866, Lexington, KY, USA - 4 December 1945, Pasadena, CA, USA, aged 79.2), American Professor at California Institute of Technology (Caltech), Pasadena, CA, USA, for his discoveries concerning the role played by the chromosome in heredity, by conducting statistical studies of the way genetic traits are passed on in fruit flies, around 1905, at the age of 39.

- The Nobel Prize in Physiology or Medicine 1983 was awarded to Barbara McClintock, 81 (16 June 1902, Hartford, CT, USA - 2 September 1992, Huntington, NY, USA, aged 90.2), American Researcher at Cold Spring Harbor Laboratory, Cold Spring Harbor, NY, USA, "for her discovery of mobile genetic elements".

1984 – Whipple, Minot, Murphy, Jerne, Köhler, Jeffreys

- 700 years ago, in 1284, eyeglasses were invented in Venice.

- 50 years ago, in 1934, the Nobel Prize in Physiology or Medicine 1934 was awarded to **George Hoyt Whipple**, 56 (28 August 1878, Ashland, NH, USA - 1 February 1976, Rochester, NY, USA, aged 97 years 5 months and 4 days), American Professor at University of Rochester, Rochester, NY, USA, **George Richards Minot**, 49 (2 December 1885, Boston, MA, USA - 25 February 1950, Brookline, MA, USA, aged 64.2), American Professor at Harvard University, Cambridge, MA, USA, and **William Parry Murphy,** 42 (6 February 1892, Stoughton, WI, USA - 9 October 1987, Brookline, MA, USA, aged 95 years 8 months and 3 days), American Lecturer at Harvard University, Cambridge, MA, USA, Peter Brent Brigham Hospital, Boston, MA, USA, "for their discoveries concerning liver therapy in cases of anaemia - at the beginning of the 1920s Whipple showed that formation of blood cells was stimulated by a diet rich in foods like liver, kidney, meat and apricots. In 1926 George Minot and William Murphy analyzed the cause of pernicious anemia, which is a shortage of a substance that later proved to be vitamin B12, which is found in liver.

- The Nobel Prize in Physiology or Medicine 1984 was awarded to **Niels K. Jerne**, 73 (23 December 1911, London, United Kingdom - 7 October 1994, Castillon-du-Gard, France, aged 82.8), British-born Swiss Researcher at Basel Institute for Immunology, Basel, Switzerland, **Georges J.F. Köhler**, 38 (17 April 1946, Munich, Germany - 1 March 1995, Freiburg im Breisgau, Germany, aged 48.9), German-born Swiss Researcher at Basel Institute for Immunology, Basel, Switzerland, and **César Milstein**, 57 (8 October 1927, Bahia Blanca, Argentina - 24 March 2002, Cambridge, United Kingdom, aged 74.4), Argentinian-born British Researcher at MRC Laboratory of Molecular Biology, Cambridge, United Kingdom, "for theories concerning the specificity in development and control of the immune system, and the discovery of the principle for production of monoclonal antibodies".

- Sir **Alec John Jeffreys**, 34 (born 9 January 1950, Oxford, UK, now age 69 years), British geneticist, developed techniques for genetic fingerprinting and DNA profiling.

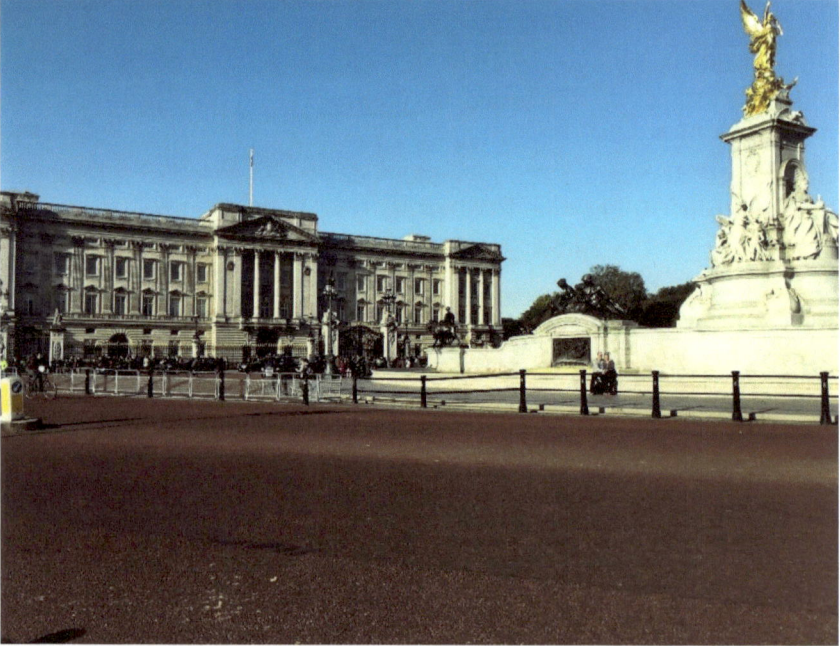

London, UK: From the Spur Rd, looking west to the Victoria Memorial (1911, 1924, right), and to the Buckingham Palace (1703, 1850, 1913, left).

1985 – i Clua, Spemann, Brown, Goldstein, Kolff

- 1 January - the Internet's Domain Name System was created.

- 100 years ago, in 1885, Spanish physician **Jaume Ferran i Clua** (1 Feb 1851 – 22 Nov 1929, aged 78.8) developed a cholera inoculation, the first to immunize humans against a bacterial disease.

- 50 years ago, in 1935, **Hugo Theorell** demonstrated how a yellow-colored enzyme in yeast had two parts, both of which were crucial to its function. He also explained how iron atoms in many enzymes have an important function in transporting electrons. He received The Nobel Prize in Physiology or Medicine 1955.

Also, in 1935, **Macfarlane Burnet** isolated a strain of influenza A virus in Australia, and subsequently did much work on serological variations of the influenza virus, and on Australian strains of the swine influenza. He received The Nobel Prize in Physiology or Medicine 1960.

Also in 1935, the Nobel Prize in Physiology or Medicine 1935 was awarded to **Hans Spemann**, 66 (27 June 1869, Stuttgart, Württemberg (now Germany) - 12 September 1941, Freiburg im Breisgau, Germany, aged 72.2), German Professor at University of Freiburg im Breisgau, Breisgau, Germany, for his discovery of the organizer effect in embryonic development - around 1920 Hans Spemann succeeded in using fine pipettes, or loops, of children's hair, to move around different parts of a frog embryo. He demonstrated that certain groups of cells adapt themselves to their surroundings while others, such as the bilaterian mouth, have an organizing effect on their surroundings. His Professor of physics in 1895 was Wilhelm Röntgen.

- The Nobel Prize in Physiology or Medicine 1985 was awarded to **Michael S. Brown**, 44 (born: 13 April 1941, New York, NY, USA), American Professor at University of Texas Southwestern Medical Center at Dallas, Dallas, TX, USA, and **Joseph L. Goldstein**,45 (born: 18 April 1940, Sumter, SC, USA),

American Professor at University of Texas Southwestern Medical Center at Dallas, Dallas, TX, USA, "for their discoveries concerning the regulation of cholesterol metabolism".

- **Willem Johan Kolff** (14 February 1911, Leiden, Netherlands – 11 February 2009, Newtown Square, PA, USA, aged 97 years 11 months and 28 days, just 3 days before 98), Dutch physician, invented the first artificial kidney dialysis machine. He also invented the first artificial kidney during WW II, and an artificial heart.

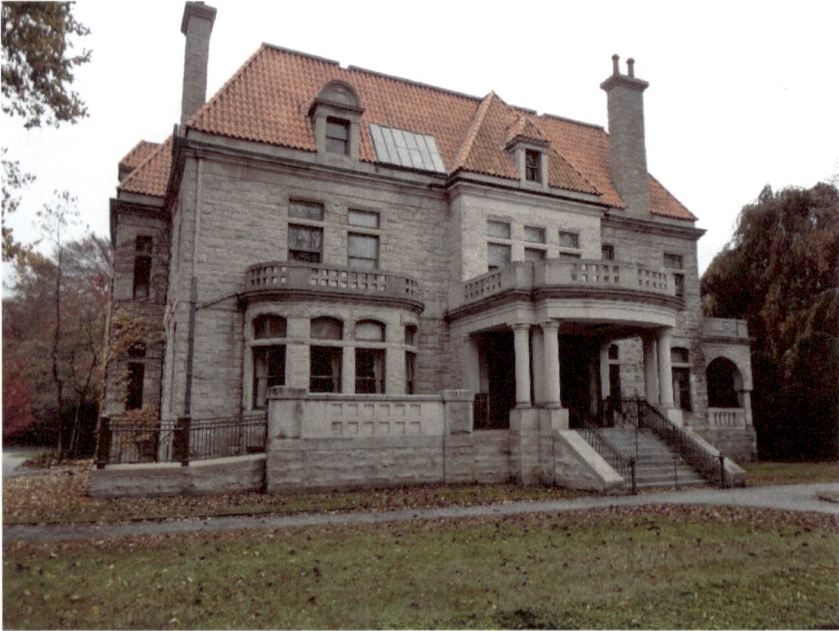

USA, Newport: Osgood-Pell House, 1888, (William H. Osgood (1830-1896, zinc)), from 1992 office for The Preservation Society of Newport County.

1986 – Fahrenheit, Dale, Loewi, Cohen, Montalcini

- 24 May - 300th anniversary of the birth of **Daniel Gabriel Fahrenheit** (24 May 1686 – 16 September 1736, aged 50.3), Dutch-German-Polish physicist, inventor, and scientific instrument maker. He invented the mercury-in-glass thermometer (first practical, accurate thermometer), and Fahrenheit scale (first standardized temperature scale to be widely used).

- 50 years ago, in 1936, the Nobel Prize in Physiology or Medicine 1936 was awarded to Sir **Henry Hallett Dale**, 61 (9 June 1875, London, United Kingdom - 23 July 1968, Cambridge, United Kingdom, aged 93 years 1 month and 14 days), British Professor at National Institute for Medical Research, London, United Kingdom, and **Otto Loewi**, 63 (3 June 1873, Frankfurt-on-the-Main, Germany - 25 December 1961, New York, NY, USA, aged 88.5), German-born Austrian Professor at Graz University, Graz, Austria, (American after 1946), for their discoveries relating to chemical transmission of nerve impulses - in 1914 Henry Dale found that acetylcholine generated stimuli in part of the nervous system, the parasympathetic nervous system, which has a dampening effect on heart activity and other functions. In 1921 Otto Loewi stimulated the heart of a frog with electrical impulses and had it pump a small amount of nutrient solution. When the fluid was transferred to another heart, it operated in a similar way. This provided proof that chemical substances convey nerve signals to organs. Otto Loewi verified the role of other substances, including acetylcholine, in this context. After Otto Loewi demonstrated acetylcholine's function as a messenger between nerves and organs, Dale and other researchers refined the understanding of acetylcholine's role in the nervous system.

- The Nobel Prize in Physiology or Medicine 1986 was awarded to **Stanley Cohen**, 64 (born: 17 November 1922, Brooklyn, NY, USA), American Professor at Vanderbilt University School of Medicine, Nashville, TN, USA, and **Rita Levi-Montalcini**, 77 (22 April 1909, Turin, Italy - 30 December 2012, Rome, Italy, aged 103 years 8 months and 8 days), Italian Researcher at Institute of Cell

Biology of the C.N.R., Rome, Italy "for their discoveries of growth factors"

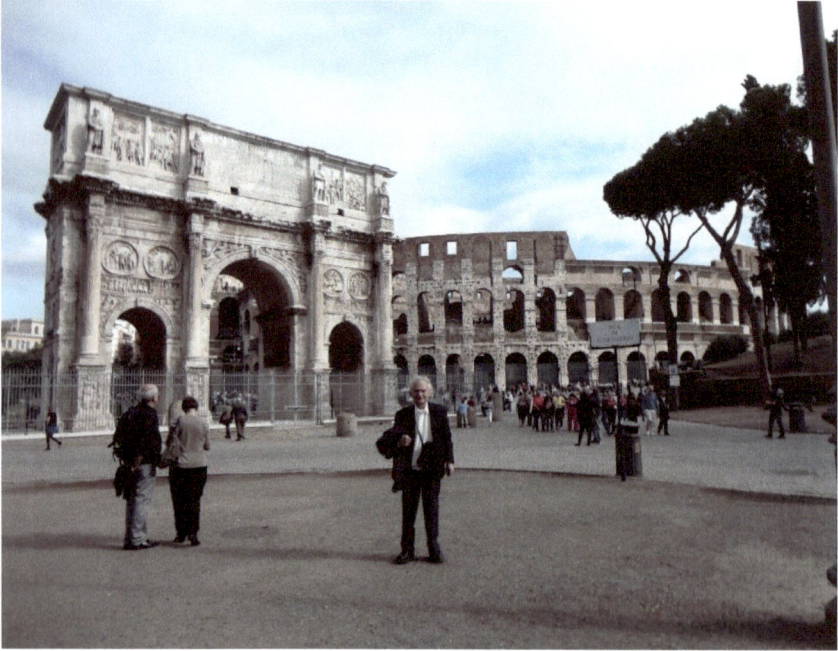

Italy, Roma: The south side of the Arch of Constantine (315, left), and the south-west side of Amphitheatrum Flavium (Colosseum, 80 AD).

1987 – Nagyrápolt, Tonegawa,

- 500 years ago, in 1487, **Leonardo da Vinci**, 35, drew L'Uomo Vitruviano (the Vitruvian Man, now at Accademia in Venice), which is regarded as a cultural icon, being reproduced on the euro coin, textbooks, etc. **Vitruvius** was an ancient Roman architect, interested in the proportions of the human body.

- 5 July - 300 years ago, in 1687, **Isaac Newton**, 44.5, published Philosophiae Naturalis Principia Mathematica.

- 100 years ago, in 1887, **F. E. Müller**, a German glassblower, made the first glass contact lenses, 379 years after Leonardo da Vinci illustrated the concept of contact lenses, in 1508.

- 50 years ago, in 1937, **Hans Krebs** (The Nobel Prize in Physiology or Medicine 1953) presented a complete picture of an important part of cell metabolism - the citric acid cycle. In this process, which is cyclical and has several steps, nutrients are converted to other molecules with a large amount of chemical energy. The latter are ultimately converted into adenosine triphosphate (ATP), which provides chemical energy to facilitate other biochemical processes in the cell.
Also, in 1937, **Daniel Bovet** (The Nobel Prize in Physiology or Medicine 1957) looked for substances that block histamines, and he found the first antihistamine, which later led to other antihistamine formulations to relieve allergies.
Also in 1937, the Nobel Prize in Physiology or Medicine 1937 was awarded to **Albert von Szent-Györgyi Nagyrápolt**, 44 (16 September 1893, Budapest, Austria-Hungary (now Hungary) - 22 October 1986, Woods Hole, MA, USA, aged 93 years 1 month and 6 days), Hungarian Professor at Szeged University, Szeged, Hungary, "for his discoveries in connection with the biological combustion processes, with special reference to vitamin C, and the catalysis of fumaric acid".

- The Nobel Prize in Physiology or Medicine 1987 was awarded to **Susumu Tonegawa**, 48 (born: 5 September 1939,

Nagoya, Japan), Japanese-born American Professor at Massachusetts Institute of Technology (MIT), Cambridge, MA, USA, "for his discovery of the genetic principle for generation of antibody diversity".

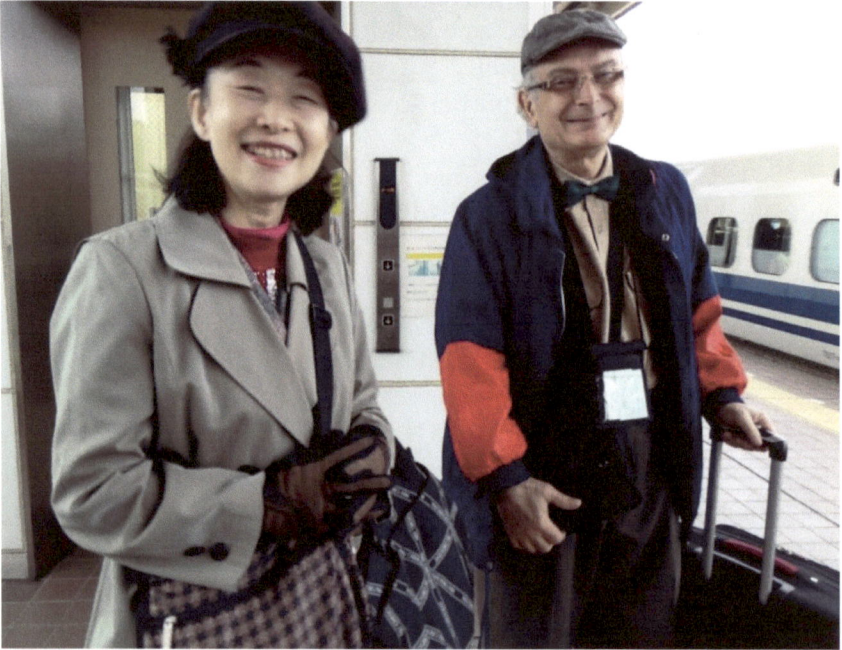

Japan, a chat with an English-speaking Japanese lady in Shin-Fuji Station, she is going to Nagoya, we are going to Kyoto.

1988 – Heymans, Black, Elion, Hitchings

- 900 years ago, in 1088, University of Bologna, Italy, was founded. It is the oldest university in continuous operation.

- 100 years ago, in 1888, The American Mathematical Society was founded.

- 50 years ago, in 1938, the Nobel Prize in Physiology or Medicine 1938 was awarded to **Corneille Jean François Heymans**, 46 (28 March 1892, Ghent, Belgium - 18 July 1968, Knokke, Belgium, aged 76.3), Belgian Professor at Ghent University, Ghent, Belgium, for the discovery of the role played by the sinus and aortic mechanisms in the regulation of respiration - in 1931 Corneille Heymans demonstrated that the glomus, a small globular body made up of small blood vessels from the carotid artery, has an important role in this context through readings of the blood's chemical composition.

- The Nobel Prize in Physiology or Medicine 1988 was awarded to Sir **James W. Black**, 64 (4 June 1924, Uddingston, Scotland - 21 March 2010, aged 85.7), British Professor at London University, King's College Hospital Medical School, London, United Kingdom, **Gertrude B. Elion**, 70 (23 January 1918, New York, NY, USA - 21 February 1999, Chapel Hill, NC, USA, aged 81), American Researcher at Wellcome Research Laboratories, Research Triangle Park, NC, USA, and **George H. Hitchings**, 83 (18 April 1905, Hoquiam, WA, USA - 27 February 1998, Chapel Hill, NC, USA, aged 92.9), American Researcher at Wellcome Research Laboratories, Research Triangle Park, NC, USA "for their discoveries of important principles for drug treatment".

1989 – Lavoisier, Domagk, Bishop, Varmus

16 March - 200th anniversary of the birth of **Georg Simon Ohm** (16 March 1789 – 6 July 1854, aged 65.3), German physicist and mathematician, who did his research with the new electrochemical cell, invented by Italian scientist Alessandro Volta. Using equipment of his own creation, Ohm found that there is a direct proportionality between the potential difference (voltage) applied across a conductor, and the resultant electric current. This relationship is known as Ohm's law.

- 200 years ago, in 1789, **Antoine Lavoisier** discovered the law of conservation of mass, the basis for chemistry, and modern chemistry begins.

- 50 years ago, in 1939, the uranium atom first split takes place at Columbia University, U.S.A.
Also, in 1939, the Nobel Prize in Physiology or Medicine 1939 was awarded to **Gerhard Domagk**, 44 (30 October 1895, Lagow, Germany (now Poland) - 24 April 1964, Burgberg, West Germany (now Germany), aged 68.5), German Professor at Munster University, Munster, Germany "for the discovery, in 1932, of the antibacterial effects of prontosil". (Gerhard Domagk was caused by the authorities of his country to decline the award, but he later received the diploma and the medal.)

- The Nobel Prize in Physiology or Medicine 1989 was awarded to **J. Michael Bishop,** 53 (born: 22 February 1936, York, PA, USA), American Professor at University of California School of Medicine, San Francisco, CA, USA, and **Harold E. Varmus**, 50 (born: 18 December 1939, Oceanside, NY, USA), American Professor at University of California School of Medicine, San Francisco, CA, USA, "for their discovery of the cellular origin of retroviral oncogenes"

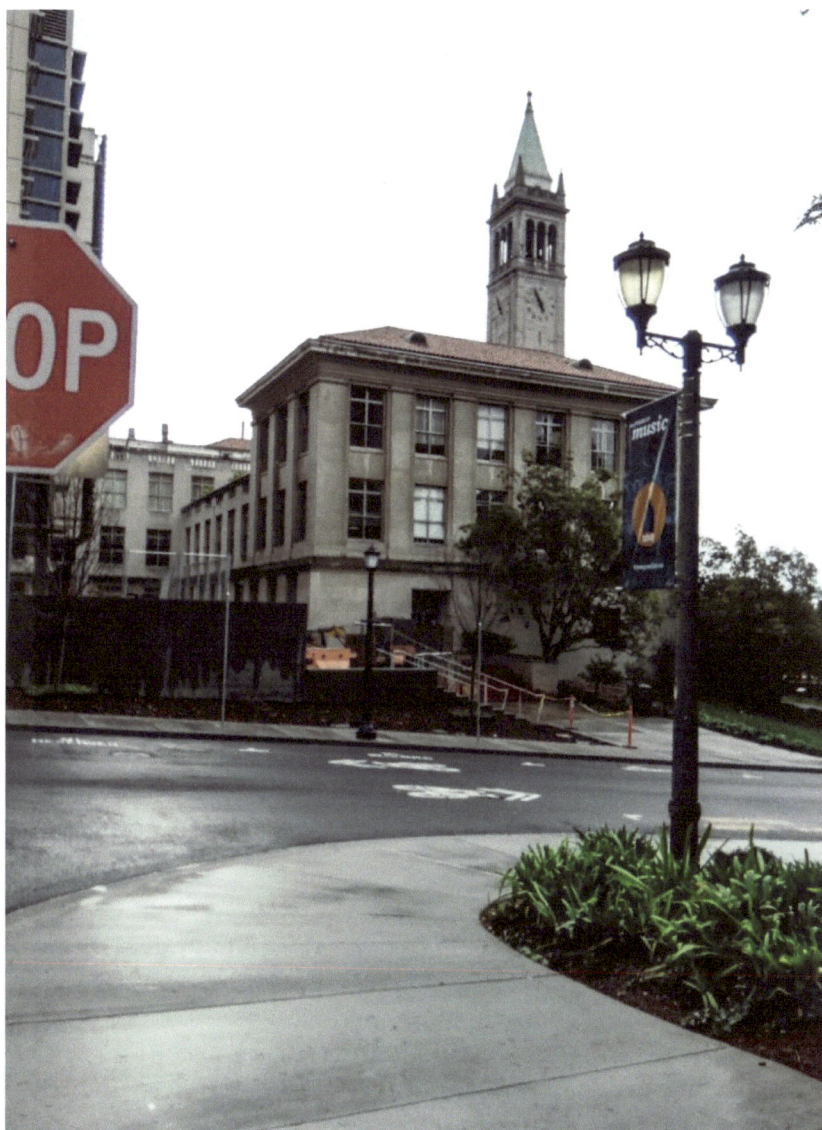

USA, the University of California, Berkeley (1868, named after the philosopher and mathematician Bishop George Berkeley (1685-1753), motto Fiat lux (Let there be light), 36,200 students, 72 Nobel laureates, 500 ha campus), Physics Department in Le Conte Hall (1924, center), Campanile (back (61 bells (full concert carillon) and clock tower). 1914, 94 m, 7 floors, observation deck on the 8th floor, inspired by il Campanile (850, 1514, 1912, 99 m) di San Marco (1084), Venezia (421, Venice), Italy (900 BC)).

1990 – Hippocrates, Dioscorides, Janssen, Blundell, Murray

- 2450th anniversary of the birth of **Hippocrates** (c. 460 BC, Island of Cos, Greece — c. 375 BC, Larissa, Thessaly, Greece, aged 85), Greek philosopher and physician, who wrote the Corpus Hippocraticum - he is the father of medicine. He began the scientific study of medicine, and prescribed a form of aspirin. Quotes:

Walking is man's best medicine.

Cure sometimes, treat often, comfort always.

Everything in excess is opposed to nature.

Extreme remedies are very appropriate for extreme diseases.

Healing is a matter of time, but it is sometimes also a matter of opportunity.

If we could give every person the right amount of nourishment and exercise, not too little and not too much, we would have found the safest way to health.

Keep a watch also on the faults of the patients, which often make them lie about the taking of things prescribed.

Let food be thy medicine, and medicine be thy food.

Life is short, the art long.

Wherever the art of medicine is loved, there is also a love of humanity.

It is more important to know what sort of person has a disease, than to know what sort of disease a person has.

There are in fact two things, science and opinion; the former begets knowledge, the latter ignorance.

Natural forces within us are the true healers of disease.

Make a habit of two things: to help; or at least to do no harm.

- 1950th anniversary of the birth of **Pedanius Dioscorides** (c. 40 Anazarbus, Cilicia, Asia Minor, Roman Empire – c. 90, aged 50), Greek physician, pharmacologist, botanist, and author of De Materia Medica, a 5-volume Greek encyclopedia about herbal medicine and related medicinal substances, that was widely read for more than 1,500 years. He was employed as a medic in the Roman army, traveled throughout the Roman Empire, and collected samples of plants. Pedanius also left a great deal of information on milk and dairy products.

- 400 years ago, in 1590, the microscope was invented by **Zacharias Janssen**, 15, (1575 – 1638, aged 63, Dutch spectacle-maker from Middelburg), and his father Hans Janssen, c. 45.

- 27 December - 200th anniversary of the birth of **James Blundell** (27 Dec 1790, London, UK – 15 Jan 1878, London, UK, aged 87 years and 19 days), English obstetrician, physiologist, teacher and physician, who, in 1818, at age 28, performed the first successful human-to-human transfusion of blood to a patient, for treatment of a haemorrhage.

- 50 years ago, in 1940, Dr. **Charles Huggins**, 39, showed that the course of the prostate cancer can be affected by hormones. If the production of male sex hormone is prevented through castration or if female sex hormone is added, the cancer could be counteracted. Hormone treatment for prostate cancer quickly gained traction. Charles Huggins also developed hormone treatment for breast cancer. He received the Nobel Prize in 1966.
Also, in 1940, no Nobel Prize was awarded.

- The Nobel Prize in Physiology or Medicine 1990 was awarded to **Joseph E. Murray**, 71 (1 April 1919, Milford, MA, USA - 26 November 2012, Boston, MA, USA, aged 93.6), American Researcher at Brigham and Women's Hospital, Boston, MA, USA, and **E. Donnall Thomas**, 70 (15 March 1920, Mart, TX, USA - 20 October 2012, Seattle, WA, USA, aged 92.6), American Researcher at Fred Hutchinson Cancer Research Center, Seattle, WA, USA, "for their discoveries concerning organ and cell transplantation in the treatment of human disease".

1991 – Pravaz, Neher, Sakmann

- 400 years ago, in 1591, the first flush toilet was introduced by Sir **John Harrington** of England, the design published under the title 'The Metamorphosis of Ajax'.

- 24 March - 200th anniversary of the birth of **Charles Gabriel Pravaz** (24 March 1791, Le Pont-de-Beauvoisin, Isère, France – 23 June 1853, Lyon, France, age 62.2), French orthopedic surgeon and inventor in 1853 (age 62) of the hypodermic syringe. While the concept dated to Galen, about 1,800 years ago, the modern syringe is thought to have originated about 500 years ago in 15th-century Italy, although it took several centuries for the device to be developed in 1853.

- 14 November - 100th anniversary of the birth of Sir **Frederick Grant Banting** (14 Nov 1891, Alliston, New Tecumseth, Canada – 21 Feb 1941, Musgrave Harbour, Canada, aged 49.2), Canadian medical scientist, physician, painter, and Nobel laureate, noted as the co-discoverer of insulin, in 1921 (age 30), and its therapeutic potential. In 1923 Banting, 32, and John James Rickard Macleod, 47, received the Nobel Prize in Medicine.

- 50 years ago, in 1941, **John Enders**, **Frederick Robbins**, and **Thomas Weller** (they received The Nobel Prize in Physiology or Medicine 1954) succeeded in culturing the virus, that causes polio in human muscle and tissue, in a laboratory setting. This became an important step on the road toward a vaccine against polio.

Also, in 1941, **George Beadle** and **Edward Tatum** (they received The Nobel Prize in Physiology or Medicine 1958) proved that our genetic code, our genes, govern the formation of enzymes. They exposed a type of mold to x-rays, causing mutations, or changes in its genes. They later succeeded in proving that this led to definite changes in enzyme formation. The conclusion was that each enzyme corresponds to a particular gene.

Also, in 1941, no Nobel Prize was awarded.

 - The Nobel Prize in Physiology or Medicine 1991 was awarded to **Erwin Neher**, 47 (born: 20 March 1944, Landsberg, Germany), German Professor at Max-Planck-Institut für Biophysikalische Chemie, Göttingen, Federal Republic of Germany, and **Bert Sakmann**, 49 (born: 12 June 1942, Stuttgart, Germany), German Professor at Max-Planck-Institut für medizinische Forschung, Heidelberg, Federal Republic of Germany, "for their discoveries concerning the function of single ion channels in cells".

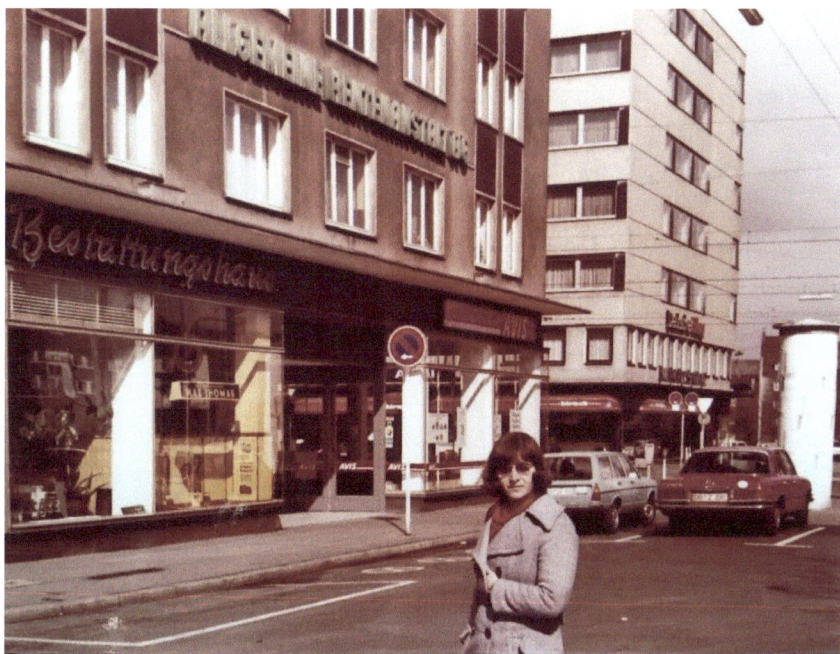

Germany, Dortmund (170 km west of Göttingen), 22 March 1978, the store Besta Hungshans (left), Avis rental service (center).

1992 – Möhring, Fischer, Krebs

- 28 October – 200 years ago, in 1792, **Paul Möhring**, German physician and botanist, died at the age of 82.3 (21 July 1710 – 28 October 1792).

- 50 years ago, in 1942, no Nobel Prize was awarded.

- The Nobel Prize in Physiology or Medicine 1992 was awarded to **Edmond H. Fischer**, 72 (born: 6 April 1920, Shanghai, China), China-born Swiss-educated American Professor at University of Washington, Seattle, WA, USA, and **Edwin G. Krebs**, 74 (6 June 1918, Lansing, IA, USA - 21 December 2009, Seattle, WA, USA, aged 91.5), American Professor at University of Washington, Seattle, WA, USA, "for their discoveries concerning reversible protein phosphorylation as a biological regulatory mechanism".

- The first vaccine was developed for hepatitis A, by Merck.

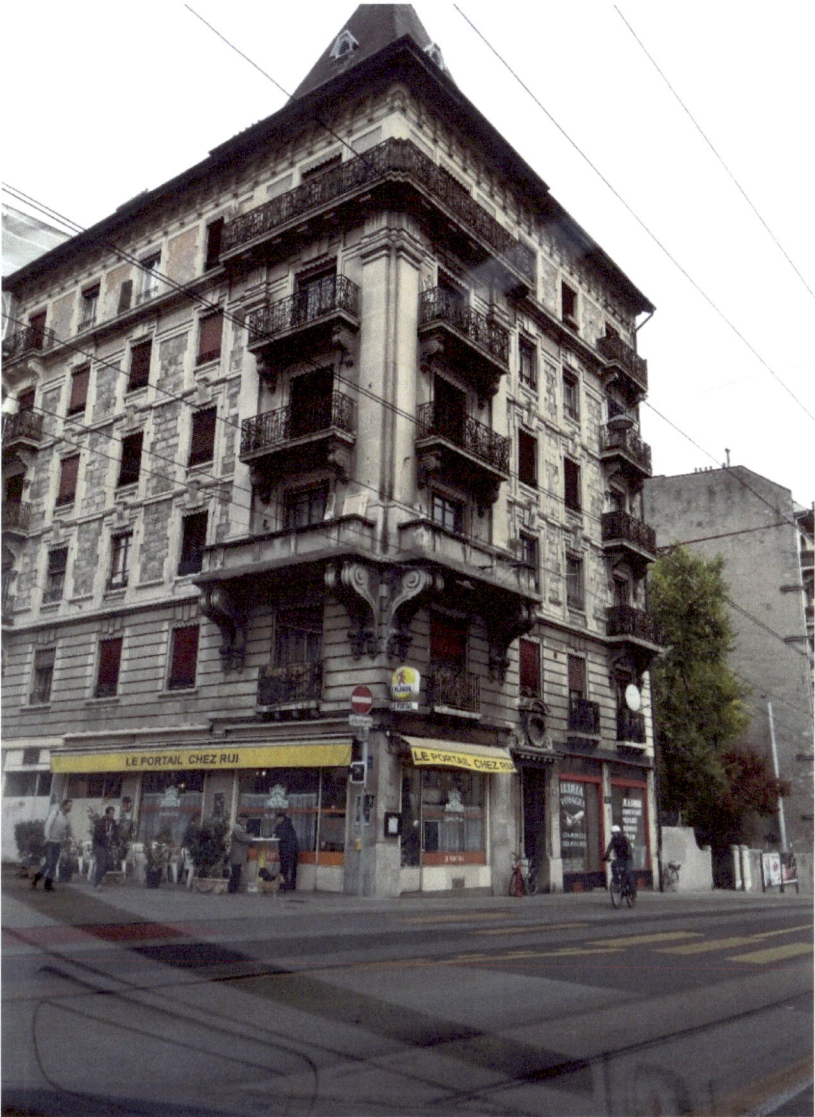

Geneva (121 BC under Romans, 375 m elevation, population 200,000, area 16 km², 70 km northwest of Mont Blanc (4810 m)), on Rue de la Servette (to the right, going southeast, Rue Jean Robert Chouet ((1642-1731, physician and politician) (the street is to the left, going northeast)), a nice building having down the restaurant Le Portail Chez Rui (yellow), 1.6 km northwest from Jet d'Eau, 1.6 km southwest from Palais des Nations (UN), 1.4 km northwest from the Université de Genève (1559, John Calvin (1509-1564)).

Chapter 6. 1993 – 2002: Imhotep, Alcmaeon, Paracelsus, Celsius, Galilei

1993 – Paracelsus, Galilei, Addison, Roberts, Sharp

- 500th anniversary of the birth of **Paracelsus** (11 November or 17 December 1493 in Einsiedeln, Switzerland – 24 September 1541 in Salzburg, Austria, aged 47.7), Swiss physician and botanist.

- 400 years ago, in 1593, **Galileo Galilei** invented the thermometer.

- April - 200th anniversary of the birth of **Thomas Addison** (April 1793 – 29 June 1860, aged 67.2), English physician and scientist.

- The Nobel Prize in Physiology or Medicine 1993 was awarded to **Richard J. Roberts**, 50 (born: 6 September 1943, Derby, United Kingdom), British-born American Researcher at New England Biolabs, Beverly, MA, USA, and **Phillip A. Sharp**, 49 (born: 6 June 1944, Falmouth, KY, USA), American Professor at Massachusetts Institute of Technology (MIT), Center for Cancer Research, Cambridge, MA, USA, "for their discoveries of split genes".

1994 – Dalton, Gilman, Rodbell

- 21 November - 300th anniversary of the birth of François-Marie Arouet (21 November 1694 – 30 May 1778, aged 83.5), known by his nom de plume **Voltaire**, a French writer, historian and philosopher famous for his wit, and his advocacy of freedom of religion, freedom of speech, and separation of church and state. Voltaire was a versatile and prolific writer, producing works in almost every literary form, including plays, poems, novels, essays, and historical and scientific works. He wrote more than 20,000 letters, and more than 2,000 books and pamphlets.

- 31 October – 200 years ago, in 1794, John Dalton, 28, (6 September 1766 – 27 July 1844, aged 77.9, English chemist, physicist, and meteorologist) delivered a ground-breaking paper on color blindness (also called Daltonism, a condition which he inherited) to the Manchester Literary and Philosophical Society in England.

- The Nobel Prize in Physiology or Medicine 1994 was awarded to **Alfred G. Gilman**, 53 (1 July 1941, New Haven, CT, USA - 23 December 2015, Dallas, TX, USA, aged 74.5), American Professor at University of Texas Southwestern Medical Center at Dallas, Dallas, TX, USA, and **Martin Rodbell**, 69 (1 December 1925, Baltimore, MD, USA - 7 December 1998, Chapel Hill, NC, USA, aged 73 years and 6 days), American Researcher at National Institute of Environmental Health Sciences, Research Triangle Park, NC, USA, "for their discovery of G-proteins and the role of these proteins in signal transduction in cells".

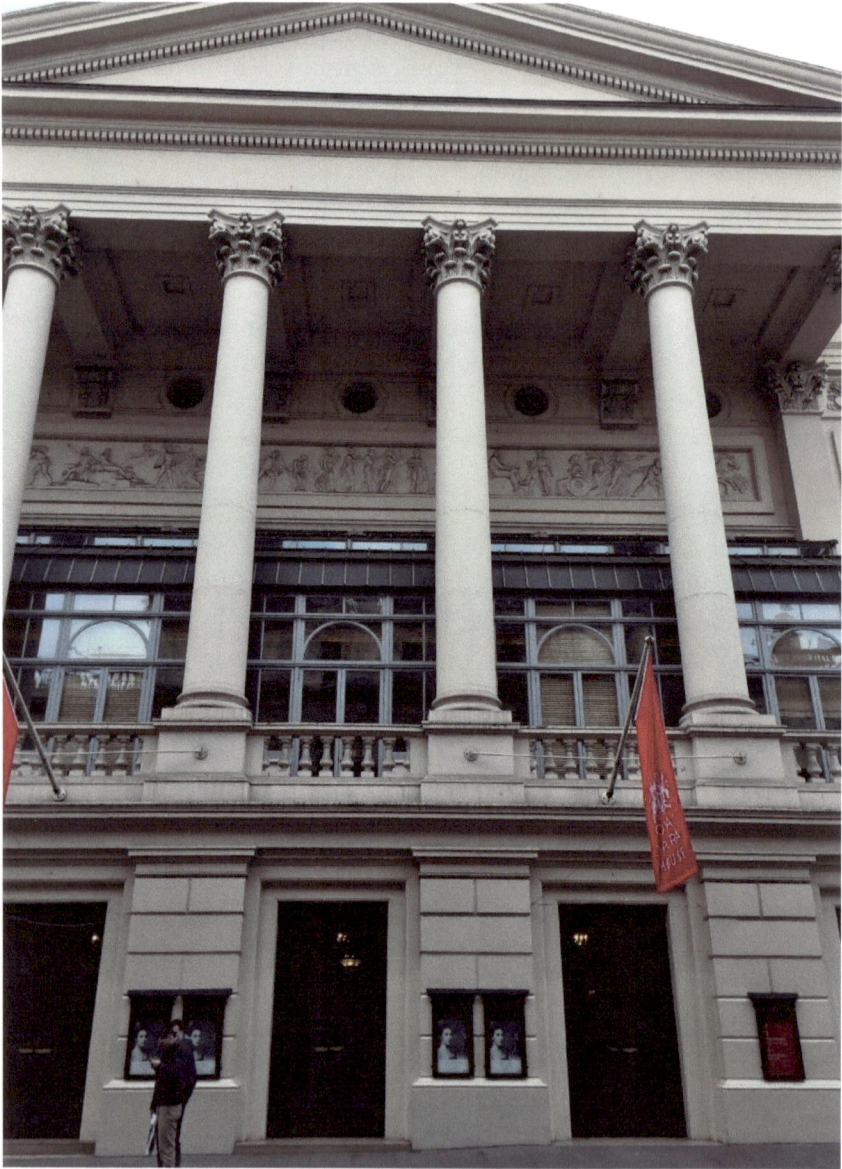

From the Bow Street, the northeast façade of the Royal Opera House at Covent Garden (1732, 1808, 1858, 1999, capacity 2,256). In 1734, Covent Garden presented its first ballet, Pygmalion. On 14 January 1947, the Covent Garden Opera Company gave its first performance of Carmen (1875, opera in four acts, based on a novella of the same title by Prosper Mérimée (1803-1870 (aged 67))) by French composer Georges Bizet (1838-1875 (aged 36)).

1995 – Blane, Röntgen, Lewis, Nüsslein-Volhard, Wieschaus

- 200 years ago, in 1795, the British Royal Navy makes the use of lemon juice mandatory to prevent scurvy, largely due to **Gilbert Blane**, 46, (29 August 1749 – 26 June 1834, aged 84.8, Scottish physician who instituted health reform in the Royal Navy).

- 100 years ago, in 1895, **Wilhelm Röntgen** identifies x-rays.

- The Nobel Prize in Physiology or Medicine 1995 was awarded to **Edward B. Lewis**, 77 (20 May 1918, Wilkes-Barre, PA, USA - 21 July 2004, Pasadena, CA, USA, aged 86.2), American Professor at California Institute of Technology (Caltech), Pasadena, CA, USA, **Christiane Nüsslein-Volhard**, 53 (born: 20 October 1942, Magdeburg, Germany), German Professor at Max-Planck-Institut für Entwicklungsbiologie, Tübingen, Federal Republic of Germany, and **Eric F. Wieschaus**, 48 (born: 8 June 1947, South Bend, IN, USA), American Professor at Princeton University, Princeton, NJ, USA, "for their discoveries concerning the genetic control of early embryonic development".

1996 – Doherty, Zinkernagel

- 14 May – 200 years ago, in 1796, **Edward Jenner**, 46.99, (17 May 1749 – 26 Jan 1823, aged 73.6, English physician and scientist) administers the first smallpox vaccination; smallpox killed an estimated 400,000 Europeans each year during the 18th century, including five reigning monarchs.

- 5 July - Dolly the sheep was cloned by **Keith Campbell**, **Ian Wilmut** and colleagues at the Roslin Institute, part of the University of Edinburgh, Scotland, and the biotechnology company PPL Therapeutics, based near Edinburgh.

- The Nobel Prize in Physiology or Medicine 1996 was awarded to **Peter C. Doherty**, 56 (born: 15 October 1940, Brisbane, Australia), Australian born American Researcher at St. Jude Children's Research Hospital, Memphis, TN, USA, and **Rolf M. Zinkernagel**, 52 (born: 6 January 1944, Basel, Switzerland), Swiss Professor at University of Zurich, Institute of Experimental Immunology, Zurich, Switzerland, "for their discoveries concerning the specificity of the cell mediated immune defence"

1997 – **Tissot, Abel, Prusiner**

- 13 June – 200 years ago, in 1797, **Samuel-Auguste Tissot**, died at the age of 69.2 (20 March 1728 – 13 June 1797), reputed Swiss neurologist, physician, professor and Vatican adviser, who practiced in Lausanne. He wrote on the diseases of the poor, men of letters and of rich people, and on nervous diseases.

- 6 May – 100 years ago, in 1897, **John Jacob Abel**, 40, (19 May 1857 – 26 May 1938, aged 81 years and 7 days, American biochemist and pharmacologist) announced the successful isolation of epinephrine (adrenaline), before the Association of American Physicians.

- The Nobel Prize in Physiology or Medicine 1997 was awarded to **Stanley B. Prusiner**, 55 (born: 28 May 1942, Des Moines, IA, USA), American Professor at University of California School of Medicine, San Francisco, CA, USA, "for his discovery of Prions – a new biological principle of infection".

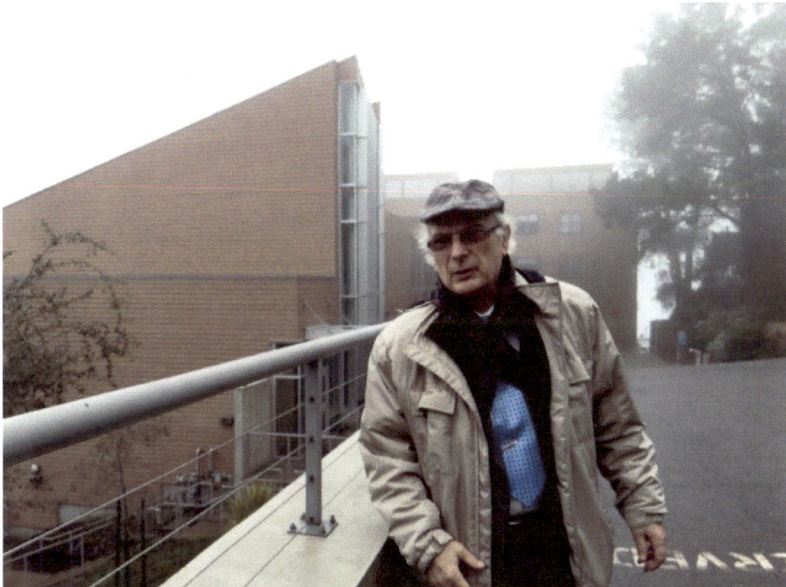

USA, University of California, Berkeley (1868), Mathematical Sciences Research Institute (1982), at 17 Gauss Way, on the hill.

1998 – Gutenberg, O'Dwyer, Furchgott, Ignarro, Murad

- 600th anniversary of the birth of **Johannes Gensfleisch zur Laden zum Gutenberg** (1398 – 3 February 1468, aged 69), known as Gutenberg, German blacksmith, goldsmith, printer, and publisher, who introduced printing to Europe with the printing press.

- 7 January – 100 years ago, in 1898, **Joseph O'Dwyer** passed away at the age of 56.2 (12 October 1841 – 7 January 1898, American physician). He developed a system of intubation in diphtheria cases.

- The Nobel Prize in Physiology or Medicine 1998 was awarded to **Robert F. Furchgott**, 82 (4 June 1916, Charleston, SC, USA - 19 May 2009, Seattle, WA, USA, aged 92.9), American Professor at SUNY Health Science Center, Brooklyn, NY, USA, **Louis J. Ignarro**, 57 (born: 31 May 1941, Brooklyn, NY, USA), American Professor at University of California School of Medicine, Los Angeles, CA, USA, and **Ferid Murad**, 62 (born: 14 September 1936, Whiting, IN, USA), American Professor at University of Texas Medical School at Houston, Houston, TX, USA, "for their discoveries concerning nitric oxide as a signalling molecule in the cardiovascular system".

<u>1999</u> – <u>Best, Blobel</u>

- 27 February – 100th anniversary of the birth of **Charles Best** (27 February 1899 – 31 March 1978, aged 79.1), American-born Canadian medical scientist, and one of the co-discoverers of insulin.

- The Nobel Prize in Physiology or Medicine 1999 was awarded to **Günter Blobel**, 63 (21 May 1936, Waltersdorf (now Niegoslawice), Germany (now Poland) - 18 February 2018, New York, NY, USA, aged 81.7), German-born American Professor at Rockefeller University, New York, NY, USA, "for the discovery that proteins have intrinsic signals that govern their transport and localization in the cell".

Günter Blobel, 63, wrote in his "Biographical" for The Nobel Prize in Physiology or Medicine 1999: "I graduated in November 1966, and decided to join George Palade's Laboratory of Cell Biology at the Rockefeller University (formerly the Rockefeller Institute). The revolution that began there in 1945, and that led to the discovery of all the major structures of the cell continued in the realm of relating cellular structures to specific cellular functions. My arrival there coincided with the end of this second phase and the exciting beginnings of a third phase, the molecular analysis of cellular functions (see below). I was fortunate enough in helping to initiate this third phase of analysis which is still in full swing.

George Palade has been my most influential mentor, a good friend and a wonderful colleague. He taught me how to conceptualize a collection of disparate facts, to formulate working hypotheses and to design experiments to test these hypotheses. I am greatly indebted to him."

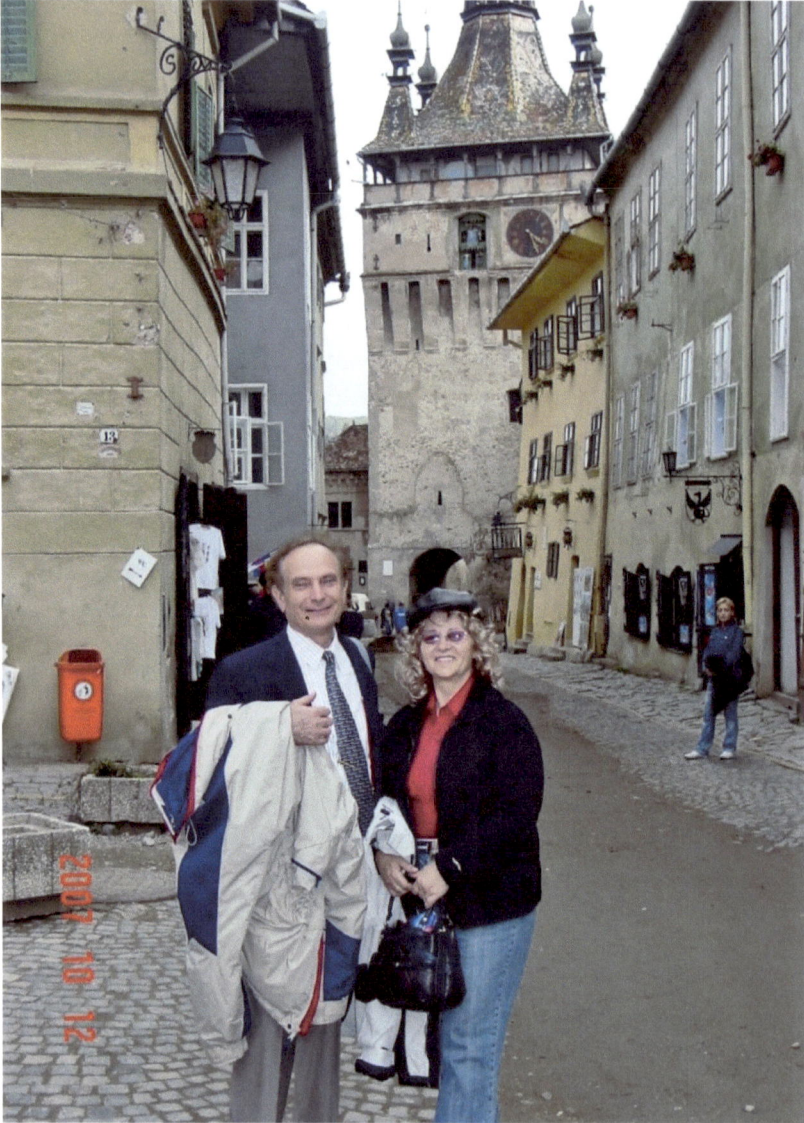

Brasov, Romania: 12 Oct 2007, a nice old street with an impressive tower above a gate. Brasov has 255,000 people living within the city, making it the 7th most populous city in Romania, and the metropolitan area is home to 370,000 residents. Braşov is located in the central part of the country, about 166 km north of Bucharest and 380 km from the Black Sea. It is surrounded by the Southern Carpathians, and is part of the Transylvania region

2000 – Imhotep, Alcmaeon of Croton, Carlsson, Greengard

- circa 4600 years ago, in circa 2600 BC, the Egyptian **Imhotep** (Greek name Imouthes, c. 2667 BC – c. 2600 BC, aged c. 67, polymath (a person expert in many areas of learning), first physician, chancellor to the second pharaoh of the 3rd dynasty during the Old Kingdom, and the founder of this epoch, Djoser (c. 2650 BC – c. 2575 BC, aged c. 75), probable first chief architect of the step pyramid built at the necropolis of Ṣaqqārah in the city of Memphis, and high priest of the Sun god Ra at Heliopolis (in the 2500 years following his death, by 100 BC, he was gradually glorified and deified, also deified by the Greeks as Asclepius, the God of healing)) described the diagnosis and treatment of about 200 diseases – he laid the foundations for the medical profession over 4600 years ago, in the 27th century BC, and was considered the God of learning and medicine. His name means 'The One Who Comes in Peace'.

- c. 2500 BC years ago, in c. 500 BC **Alcmaeon of Croton** (c. 540 BC – 500 BC, aged 40, Greek Presocratic philosopher and physiologist of the Academy at Croton (Greek city-state in Magna Graecia, now Crotone, southern Italy), medical writer of antiquity, first to practice dissection for research purposes), distinguished veins from arteries.

- The Nobel Prize in Physiology or Medicine 2000 was awarded to **Arvid Carlsson**, 77 (25 January 1923, Uppsala, Sweden - 29 June 2018, Gothenburg, Sweden, aged 95.4), Swedish Professor at Göteborg University, Gothenburg, Sweden, **Paul Greengard**, 75 (born: 11 December 1925, New York, NY, USA), American Professor at Rockefeller University, New York, NY, USA, and **Eric R. Kandel**, 71 (born: 7 November 1929, Vienna, Austria), Austrian-born American Professor at Columbia University, New York, NY, USA, "for their discoveries concerning signal transduction in the nervous system".

2001 – Celsius, von Behring, Röntgen, Hartwell, Hunt, Nurse

- 2001 is the 1st year of the 3rd millennium, and the 1st year of the 21st century.

- 27 November – 300th anniversary of the birth of **Anders Celsius** (27 November 1701 – 25 April 1744, aged 42.4), Swedish mathematician, astronomer, and physicist. He founded the Uppsala Astronomical Observatory in 1741, and in 1742 proposed the Celsius temperature scale, which bears his name.

- 100 years ago, in 1901, when the 20th century began, German physiologist **Emil von Behring**, 47 (15 March 1854, Hansdorf (now Lawice), Prussia (now Poland) - 31 March 1917, Marburg, Germany, aged 63; he had six sons), German Professor at Marburg University, Marburg, Germany, received the 1901 Nobel Prize in Physiology or Medicine, the first one awarded, for his discovery of a diphtheria antitoxin - in 1900 Emil von Behring introduced serum from immune horses as a method to cure and prevent diphtheria. In 1888, he, 34, worked as an assistant at the Institute of Hygiene, under Robert Koch, 45. He remained there for several years after 1889, and followed Koch when the latter moved to the Institute for Infectious Diseases.

- 100 years ago, in 1901, **Wilhelm Conrad Röntgen**, 56, German mechanical engineer and physicist, who, on 8 November 1895, at age 50.6, produced and detected electromagnetic radiation in a wavelength range known as X-rays or Röntgen rays, received the first Nobel Prize in Physics.

- The Nobel Prize in Physiology or Medicine 2001 was awarded to **Leland H. Hartwell**, 62 (born: 30 October 1939, Los Angeles, CA, USA), American Researcher at Fred Hutchinson Cancer Research Center, Seattle, WA, USA, **Tim Hunt**, 58 (born: 19 February 1943, Neston, United Kingdom), British Researcher at Imperial Cancer Research Fund, London, United Kingdom, and Sir **Paul M. Nurse**, 52 (born: 25 January 1949, Norwich, United Kingdom), British Researcher at Imperial Cancer Research Fund,

London, United Kingdom, "for their discoveries of key regulators of the cell cycle".

Note: Sir Paul M. Nurse, 52, wrote at the beginning of his "Biographical" for The Nobel Prize in Physiology or Medicine 2001: "My parents were born in Norfolk and spent their early years working in the big houses of that rural English county, my mother as a cook and my father as a handyman and chauffeur. After the 1930s recession they moved to Wembley, North-West London, where my father worked as a mechanic in the local H.J. Heinz food processing factory, and my mother brought up their four children and was a part-time cleaner. I was by far the youngest of the family, and at times it was like being an only child. My parents were neither wealthy nor academic, but we lived comfortably and they were always extremely supportive of my academic efforts and aspirations, both at school and university."

Then Sir Paul M. Nurse, 59, added "Addendum, February 2008": It was six years after these words were written when I was 57 years of age, that I discovered my parents were not my parents. This revelation came about because of the US Department of Homeland Security rejecting my Green Card application on the grounds that the details given on my birth certificate were insufficient. In the UK there is both a short and a long birth certificate, and the former which I had did not record the names of parents. I applied to the UK Registry Office for a long certificate and went on holiday. On my return, I was greeted by my PA asking if "I had made a mistake with the name of my mother." She handed me the new long birth certificate and the next few seconds of my life were both unexpected and transforming. The name of my mother given on the certificate was the name of the person I thought was my sister and the space for my father's name was blank. I had been brought up by my grandparents thinking that they were my parents.

Both my mother and grandparents died some years ago so I could not confirm with them what had happened. A more distant relative had been 12 years of age and lived in the house where I was born, and had been sworn to secrecy about my birth. She was able to tell me that my mother became pregnant at 18 years and was sent away to her aunt's for the last months of pregnancy and my birth. My grandmother then came and pretended that she was the mother and returned to the family home with her "new son." My grandparents then brought me up to protect their daughter. My mother got married when I was nearly three and there is a poignant photograph of the wedding with her holding her new husband with one hand and me with her other hand. Everyone kept the secret so even my two brothers (now my uncles) did not know the truth of my origins. And of course, I still do not know who my father is beyond a rumour that he may have been a serviceman, perhaps even an American serviceman which would presumably please the US Department of Homeland Security.

Does any of this change anything? Not really, I was brought up by loving grandparents and had a happy childhood. All my relations have changed of course, with parents becoming grandparents, brothers becoming uncles, nephews and nieces becoming half brothers and sisters. In fact, it was quite nice to acquire new half siblings at a late stage in life. Both my grandparents were also illegitimate so I inherited the name 'Nurse' twice through the maternal line in three generations: so apart from being somewhat unsettled, which I suppose is understandable, nothing really has changed, although I continue to wonder who my father is. Of course, I regret not having had time with my real mother or the opportunity to discuss my origins with her later in life, and then there is the final irony that even though I am a geneticist my family managed to keep my genetic origins secret from me for over half a century.

2002 – Ross, Brenner, Horvitz, Sulston

- 100 years ago, in 1902, **Willis Carrier**, 26, invents the first modern electrical air conditioning unit.

- 100 years ago, in 1902, the Nobel Prize in Physiology or Medicine 1902 was awarded to **Ronald Ross**, 45 (13 May 1857, Almora, India (son of an English general) - 16 September 1932, Putney Heath, United Kingdom, aged 75.3), British Professor at University College, Liverpool, United Kingdom, "for his work on malaria, by which he has shown how it enters the organism and thereby has laid the foundation for successful research on this disease and methods of combating it". He was interested in mathematics, poetry and music. He created mathematical models for how the disease is spread, something that became a useful tool for epidemiology. Ronald Ross had mosquitos suck blood from malaria-infected people, and in 1897 he found the malaria parasite at a certain stage of life in the stomach of a certain species of mosquito.

- The Nobel Prize in Physiology or Medicine 2002 was awarded to **Sydney Brenner**, 75 (born 13 January 1927, Germiston, South Africa), South Africa-born American Researcher at The Molecular Sciences Institute, Berkeley, CA, USA), **H. Robert Horvitz**, 55 (born 8 May 1947, Chicago, IL, USA), American Professor at Massachusetts Institute of Technology (MIT), Cambridge, MA, USA, and **John E. Sulston**, 60 (27 March 1942, Cambridge, United Kingdom - 6 March 2018, aged 75.9), British Researcher at The Wellcome Trust Sanger Institute, Cambridge, United Kingdom, "for their discoveries concerning genetic regulation of organ development and programmed cell death"'.

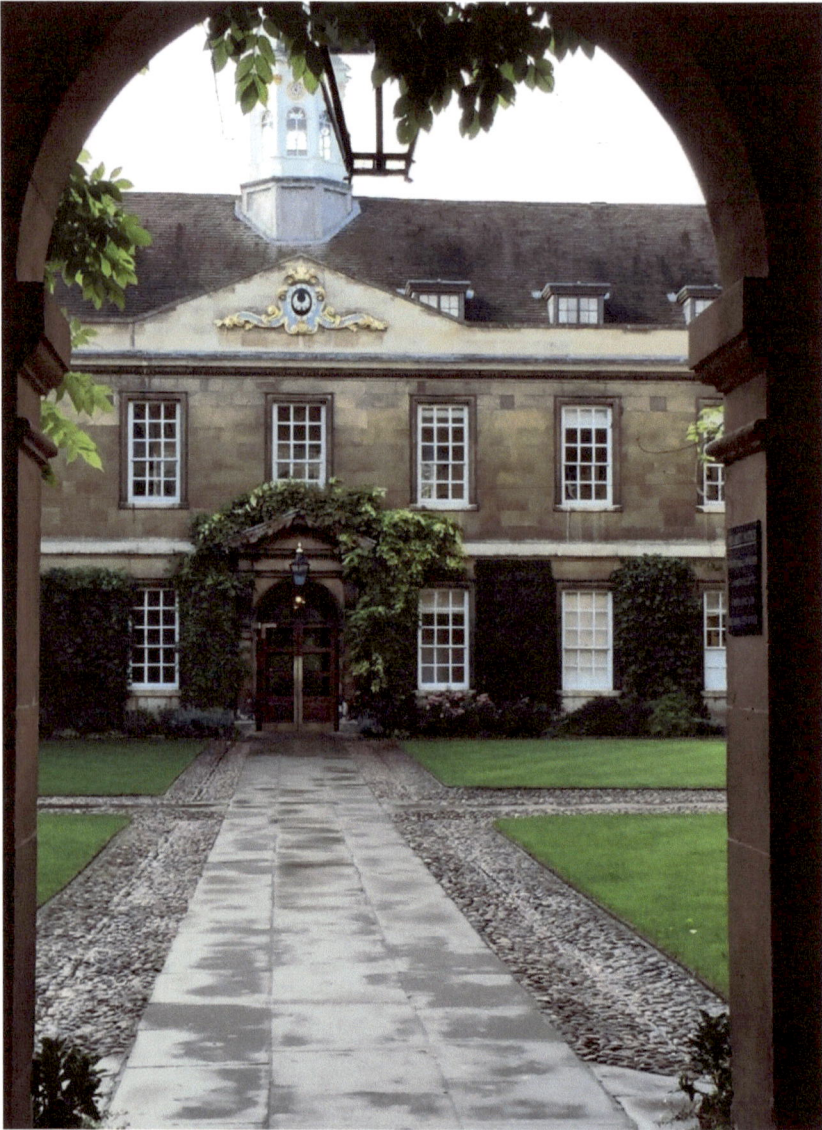

Cambridge, UK: From Trinity Ln, looking west through the entrance of Trinity Hall, (1350, by William Baterman (c 1298-1355, Bishop of Norwich between 1344 and 1355), a constituent college (the 5th oldest) of the University of Cambridge), to the Front Court and the entrance to the west building of the Front Court. To the northeast of Trinity Hall there is the separate Trinity College (1546, founder Henry VIII (1491-1547, reign 1509-1547), motto: Virtus Vera Nobilitas).

Chapter 7. 2003 – 2012: Rhazes, Darwin, Parkinson, Ehrlich

2003 – Gorrie, Finsen, Lauterbur, Mansfield

- 400 years ago, in 1603, Accademia Nazionale dei Lincei was founded in Rome, Italy (the author was invited here in 1977).

- 3 October - 200th anniversary of the birth of **John Gorrie** (3 October 1803 – 29 June 1855, aged 51.7), American physician, scientist, and inventor of mechanical cooling.

- 100 years ago, in 1903, the Nobel Prize in Physiology or Medicine 1903 was awarded to **Niels Ryberg Finsen**, 43 (15 December 1860, Thorshavn, Faroe Islands (Denmark) - 24 September 1904, Copenhagen, Denmark, aged 43.7), Danish Professor at Finsen Medical Light Institute, Copenhagen, Denmark, "in recognition of his contribution to the treatment of diseases, especially lupus vulgaris, with concentrated light radiation, whereby he has opened a new avenue for medical science". Niels Finsen suffered from a metabolic disease (which turned out to be Pick's disease) that caused weakness and fatigue, but he noticed that light made him feel more energetic. This led him to study the medical benefits of light. Soon he had a research institute of his own. In 1895 he used concentrated beams of ultraviolet light to treat patients with lupus vulgaris with some success. For a time, light therapy was widespread, but eventually it was supplanted by antibiotics.

- The Nobel Prize in Physiology or Medicine 2003 was awarded to **Paul C. Lauterbur**, 74 (6 May 1929, Sidney, OH, USA - 27 March 2007, Urbana, IL, USA, aged 77.9), Professor at University of Illinois, Urbana, IL, USA, and Sir **Peter Mansfield**, 70 (9 October 1933, London, United Kingdom - 8 February 2017, aged 83.3), British Professor at University of Nottingham, School of Physics and Astronomy, Nottingham, United Kingdom, "for their discoveries concerning magnetic resonance imaging".

2004 – Scarpa, Pavlov, Axel, Buck

- 200 years ago, in 1804, **Antonio Scarpa**, 52, ((9 May 1752 – 31 October 1832, aged 80.4), Italian anatomist and professor), published "Riflessioni ed Osservazione anatomico-chirugiche sull' Aneurisma", a classic text on aneurisms.

- 200 years ago, in 1804, the world population reached 1 billion, and the first steam locomotive begins operation.

- 100 years ago, in 1904, the Nobel Prize in Physiology or Medicine 1904 was awarded to **Ivan Petrovich Pavlov**, 55 (14 September 1849, Ryazan, Russia - 27 February 1936, Leningrad, Russia, aged 86.3), Russian Professor at the Military Medical Academy, St. Petersburg, Russia, in recognition of his work on the physiology of digestion, through which knowledge on vital aspects of the subject has been transformed and enlarged - during the 1890s he identified ways in which different parts of the body, through the nervous system, affect movements in the intestinal canal as well as secretion of gastric juice and other secretions. He also pointed out the significance of psychic factors, such as hunger's ability to activate secretion of gastric juice. Furthermore, he demonstrated the sensitivity of gastric mucosae to various chemical substances.

- The Nobel Prize in Physiology or Medicine 2004 was awarded to Richard Axel, 58 (born: 2 July 1946, New York, NY, USA), American Professor at Columbia University, New York, NY, USA, and Linda B. Buck, 57 (born: 29 January 1947, Seattle, WA, USA), American Researcher at Fred Hutchinson Cancer Research Center, Seattle, WA, USA, "for their discoveries of odorant receptors and the organization of the olfactory system".

2005 – Parkinson, Koch, Marshall, Warren

- 200 years ago, in 1805, **James Parkinson**, 50, ((11 April 1755 – 21 December 1824, aged 69.6), English surgeon, apothecary, geologist, and paleontologist, who is best known for his 1817 work, at age 62, "An Essay on the Shaking Palsy" in which he was the first to describe "paralysis agitans", later renamed Parkinson's disease by Jean-Martin Charcot) published "Observations on the Nature and Cure of the Gout".

- 100 years ago, in 1905, the Nobel Prize in Physiology or Medicine 1905 was awarded to **Robert Koch**, 62 (11 December 1843, Clausthal (now Clausthal-Zellerfeld), Germany - 27 May 1910, Baden-Baden, Germany, aged 66.4), German Professor at Institute for Infectious Diseases, Berlin, Germany, "for his investigations and discoveries in relation to tuberculosis - Robert Koch, who had conducted a range of important studies on illnesses caused by microorganisms, discovered and described the TB bacterium in 1882. He later studied tuberculin, a substance formed by tubercle bacteria.

- The Nobel Prize in Physiology or Medicine 2005 was awarded to **Barry J. Marshall**, 54 (born: 30 September 1951, Kalgoorlie, Australia), Australian Professor at NHMRC Helicobacter pylori Research Laboratory, QEII Medical Centre, Nedlands, Australia, University of Western Australia, Perth, Australia, and **J. Robin Warren**, 68 (born: 11 June 1937, Adelaide, Australia), Australian Researcher, "for their discovery of the bacterium *Helicobacter pylori* and its role in gastritis and peptic ulcer disease".

2006 – Franklin, Golgi, Cajal, Fire, Mello, Frazer, Zhou

- 17 January – 300th anniversary of the birth of **Benjamin Franklin** (January 17, 1706 – April 17, 1790, aged 84 years and 3 months), an American polymath and one of the Founding Fathers of the United States. Franklin was a leading author, printer, political theorist, politician, freemason, postmaster, scientist, inventor, humorist, civic activist, statesman, and diplomat. As a scientist he is known for his discoveries and theories regarding electricity. As an inventor, he is known for the lightning rod, bifocals (very useful for medical applications), and the Franklin stove, among other inventions. He founded many civic organizations, including Philadelphia's fire department and the University of Pennsylvania.

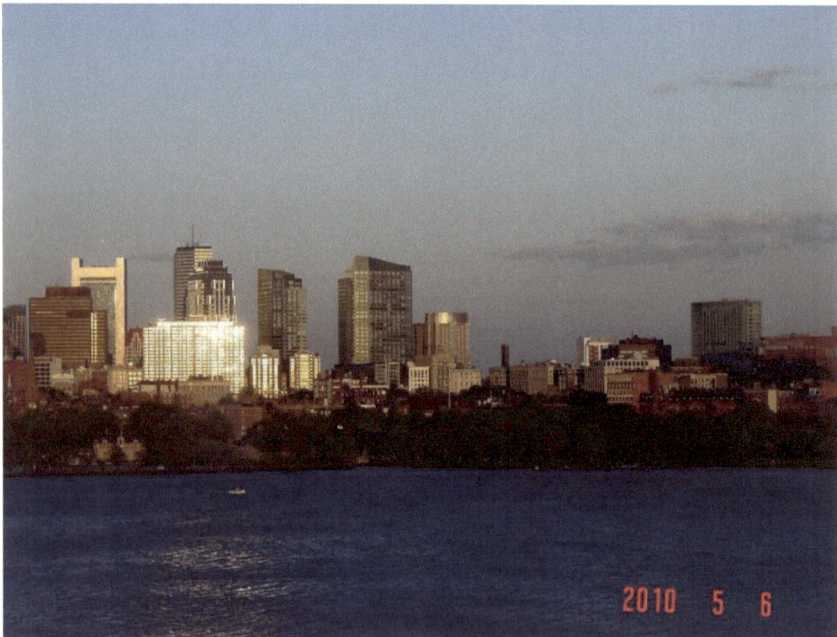

USA, Boston: a view of the north-east part of Boston, from Cambridge, over Charles River Basin. Federal Reserve Bank Building (187 m, left), and other tall buildings in the financial district.

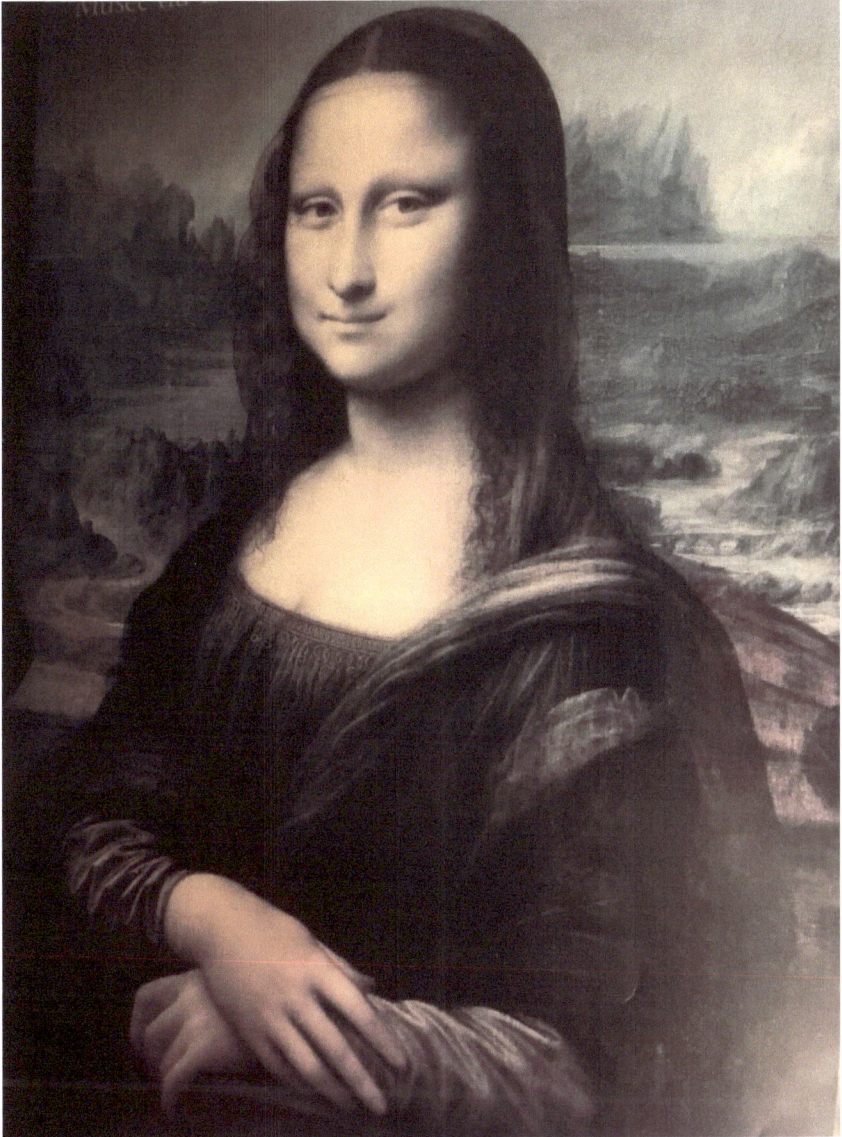

Copy of Mona Lisa (or La Gioconda, detail), 1506, by Leonardo da Vinci, 54.

- 100 years ago, in 1906, the Nobel Prize in Physiology or Medicine 1906 was awarded to **Camillo Golgi**, 63 (7 July 1843, Corteno, Italy - 21 January 1926, Pavia, Italy, aged 82.5), Italian Professor at Pavia University, Pavia, Italy, and **Santiago Ramón y Cajal**, 54 (1 May 1852, Petilla de Aragón, Spain - 17 October 1934,

Madrid, Spain, aged 82.5; he had seven children), Spanish Professor at Madrid University, Madrid, Spain, in recognition of their work on the structure of the nervous system - in the 1870s Camillo Golgi discovered that nerve cells could be stained with silver nitrate. This led to groundbreaking studies of how the nervous system is structured and functions. Santiago Ramón y Cajal began using Golgi's method in 1887, and achieved many groundbreaking results in the years that followed. This included proving that each nerve cell is an independent entity, and nerve synapses transfer nerve impulses from one cell to another.

The Nobel Prize in Physiology or Medicine 2006 was awarded to **Andrew Z. Fire**, 47 (born: 27 April 1959, Stanford, CA, USA), American Professor at Stanford University School of Medicine, Stanford, CA, USA, and **Craig C. Mello**, 46 (born: 19 October 1960, New Haven, CT, USA), American Professor at University of Massachusetts Medical School, Worcester, MA, USA, "for their discovery of RNA interference – gene silencing by double-stranded RNA".

- **Ian Hector Frazer**, 53, (born 6 January 1953), Scottish-born Australian immunologist, and Dr. **Jian Zhou** (1957 – 1999, aged 42), Chinese virologist and cancer researcher, invented Gardasil and Cervarix at the University of Queensland, the vaccines for stimulating human immunological resistance to the cervical cancer-inducing human papilloma virus (HPV).

2007 – Hahnemann, Laveran, Capecchi, Evans, Smithies

- 200 years ago, in 1807, **Samuel Hahnemann**, 52, (10 April 1755 – 2 July 1843, aged 88.2), German physician who first introduced the term 'homeopathy' in an essay.

- 100 years ago, in 1907, the Nobel Prize in Physiology or Medicine 1907 was awarded to **Charles Louis Alphonse Laveran**, 62 (18 June 1845, Paris, France - 18 May 1922, Paris, France, aged 76 years and 11 months), French Researcher at Institut Pasteur, Paris, France, in recognition of his work on the role played by protozoa in causing diseases - after examining blood from people infected with malaria, Alphonse Laveran, 44, in 1889, was able to show that malaria is caused by another type of single-celled organism, a protozoan of the Plasmodium family, which attacks red blood cells. He also identified other single-celled parasites that cause other diseases.

The Nobel Prize in Physiology or Medicine 2007 was awarded to **Mario R. Capecchi**, 70 (born: 6 October 1937, Verona, Italy), Italian-born American Professor at University of Utah, Salt Lake City, UT, USA), Sir **Martin J. Evans**, 66 (born: 1 January 1941, Stroud, United Kingdom), British Professor at Cardiff University, Cardiff, United Kingdom, and **Oliver Smithies**, 82 (23 June 1925, Halifax, United Kingdom - 10 January 2017, Chapel Hill, NC, USA, aged 91.6), British-born American Professor at University of North Carolina, Chapel Hill, NC, USA, "for their discoveries of principles for introducing specific gene modifications in mice by the use of embryonic stem cells".

2008 – von Oppolzer, Ehrlich, Mechnikov, Hausen

- 4 August - 200th anniversary of the birth of **Johann Ritter von Oppolzer** ((4 August 1808 – 16 April 1871, aged 62.6), Austrian physician, foreign member of the Royal Swedish Academy of Science.

- 100 years ago, in 1908, the German physician, bacteriologist, and chemist **Paul Ehrlich**, 54 (14 March 1854, Strehlen (now Strzelin), Prussia (now Poland) - 20 August 1915, Bad Homburg vor der Höhe, Germany, of a second stroke, aged 61.4), German Professor at Göttingen University, Göttingen, Germany, Königliches Institut für experimentelle Therapie (Royal Institute for Experimental Therapy), Frankfurt-on-the-Main, Germany, shared with **Ilya Ilyich Mechnikov**, 63 (15 May 1845, Kharkov, Russian Empire - 15 July 1916, Paris, France, of heart attacks, aged 71 years and 2 months), Russian-born French Researcher at Institut Pasteur, Paris, France, the Nobel Prize in Physiology or Medicine 1908, for their contributions to immunity - one of Paul Ehrlich's contributions to immunology was the transfer of blood serum with antibodies to treat and counteract diphtheria, which he carried out with Emil von Behring. In 1890 Robert Koch, 47, Director of the newly established Institute for Infectious Diseases, appointed Ehrlich, 36, as one of his assistants and Ehrlich then began the immunological studies with which his name will always be associated. In 1882 Mechnikov showed that phagocytosis is one of the immune system's ways of operating, that is certain cells in the blood, white blood cells, work by encapsulating and destroying harmful bacteria and other microorganisms. In 1888, Mechnikov, 43, left Odessa and went to Paris to ask Pasteur, 66, for his advice. Pasteur gave him a laboratory and an appointment in the Pasteur Institute. Here he remained for the rest of his life.

- The Nobel Prize in Physiology or Medicine 2008 was awarded to **Harald zur Hausen**, 72 (born: 11 March 1936, Gelsenkirchen, Germany), German Researcher at German Cancer Research Center, Heidelberg, Germany, "for his discovery of human papilloma viruses causing cervical cancer", and Françoise Barré-

Sinoussi, 61 (born: 30 July 1947, Paris, France), French Researcher at Regulation of Retroviral Infections Unit, Virology Department, Institut Pasteur, Paris, France, and Luc Montagnier, 76 (born: 18 August 1932, Chabris, France), "for their discovery of human immunodeficiency virus".

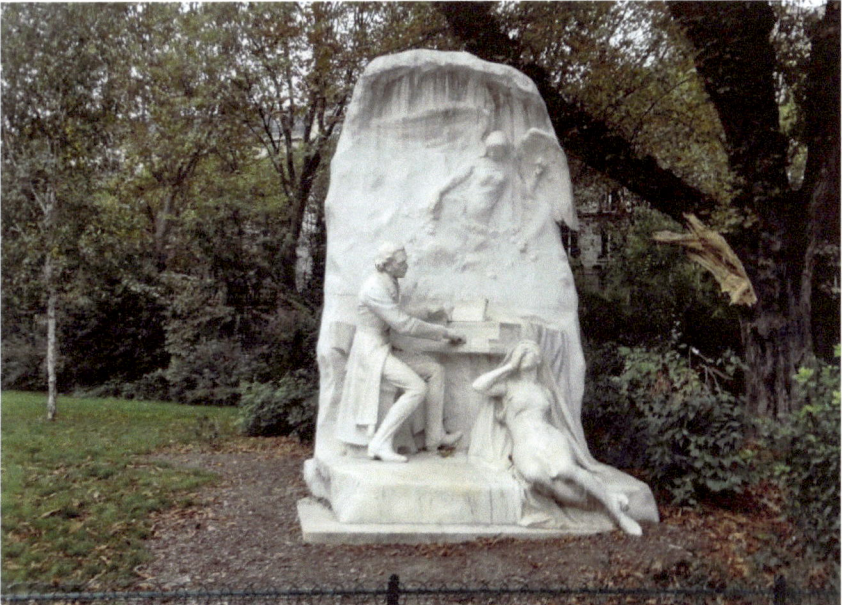

Paris, France: Monument to Frédéric Chopin (1810-1849, composer) in Parc Monceau (1779, 8.2 ha), on Boulevard de Courcelles.

<u>2009</u> – **Darwin**, **Kocher**, **Blackburn, Greider, Szostak**

- 12 February - 200th anniversary of the birth of **Charles Robert Darwin**, (12 February 1809 – 19 April 1882, aged 73.2), English naturalist, geologist and biologist, best known for his contributions to the evolution theory. He had 10 children.

- 100 years ago, in 1909, the Nobel Prize in Physiology or Medicine 1909 was awarded to **Emil Theodor Kocher**, 68 (25 August 1841, Berne, Switzerland - 27 July 1917, Berne, Switzerland, aged 75.9), Swiss Professor at Berne University, Berne, Switzerland, "for his work on the physiology, pathology and surgery of the thyroid gland - in 1883, Theodor Kocher, 42, explained the thyroid gland's function in metabolism, among other things, and showed how surgery could be carried out more safely through good hygiene, and minimal blood loss. He also showed that a viable part of the gland needs to be left intact during the operation.

- The Nobel Prize in Physiology or Medicine 2009 was awarded to Elizabeth H. Blackburn, 61 (born: 26 November 1948, Hobart, Tasmania, Australia), Australia-born American Professor at University of California, San Francisco, CA, USA, Carol W. Greider, 48, (born: 15 April 1961, San Diego, CA, USA), American Professor at Johns Hopkins University School of Medicine, Baltimore, MD, USA, and Jack W. Szostak, 57 (born: 9 November 1952, London, United Kingdom), British-born American Professor at Harvard Medical School, Boston, MA, USA, Massachusetts General Hospital, Boston, MA, USA, Howard Hughes Medical Institute, "for the discovery of how chromosomes are protected by telomeres and the enzyme telomerase".

2010 – Rhazes, Kossel, Edwards

- 1100 years ago, in 910, Persian physician and mathematician **Rhazes**, 56, (854 – 15 Oct 925, aged 71) identified smallpox. He wrote over 200 papers, some of which had an impact on European medicine.

- 100 years ago, in 1910, the Nobel Prize in Physiology or Medicine 1910 was awarded to **Albrecht Kossel**, 57 (16 September 1853, Rostock, Mecklenburg (now Germany) - 5 July 1927, Heidelberg, Germany, aged 73.7), German Professor at University of Heidelberg, Heidelberg, Germany, in recognition of the contributions to our knowledge of cell chemistry made through his work on proteins, including the nucleic substances - between 1885 and 1901, Albrecht Kossel discovered that the nucleic acids were composed of five nitrogen bases: adenine, cytosine, guanine, thymine, and uracil.

- The Nobel Prize in Physiology or Medicine 2010 was awarded to **Robert G. Edwards**, 85 (27 Sep 1925, Batley, UK – 10 April 2013, Cambridge, UK, aged 87.6), British Professor at University of Cambridge, Cambridge, United Kingdom, "for the development of in vitro fertilization" in 1978 (age 53).

The article "Spatio-Temporal Speckle Reduction in Ultrasound Sequences" by Noura Azzabou and Nikos Paragios, was published in Inverse Problems and Imaging, 4, 2, 2010, 211–222, and the author's review of this article was published, in 2010, in the Mathematical Reviews of the American Mathematical Society. In the health-care industry, the **medical analysis** of the dynamical behavior of organs is of great importance, and a practical low cost and non-invasive technique for this purpose is the **ultrasound imaging.** The technical problem is that the images that are produced receive a multiplicative component, which is the speckle. The physicians find very good information in the ultrasound image, however, the diagnosis is sometimes problematical because of this speckle, which negatively impacts the image quality. Naturally, many authors proposed methods for speckle suppression, while maintaining all image details.

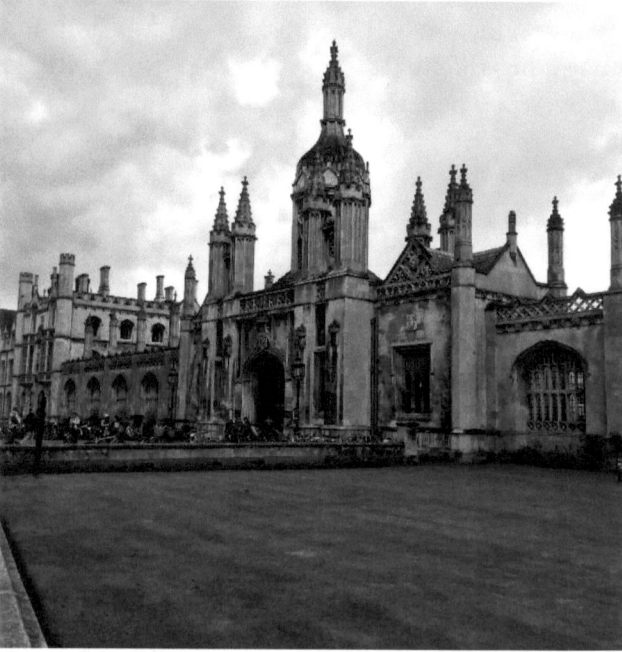

Cambridge, UK: From the King's Parade, looking southwest to the east façade of the entrance of King's College (1441, by King Henry VI (1421-1471)).

2011 – Bell, Gullstrand, Beutler, Hoffmann, Steinman

- 200 years ago, in 1811, **Charles Bell**, 37, ((12 November 1774 – 28 April 1842, aged 67.4), Scottish surgeon, anatomist, physiologist and neurologist), published "An Idea of a New Anatomy of the Brain", distinguishing between sensory and motor nerves in the spinal cord. He also described Bell's palsy.

- 100 years ago, in 1911, the Nobel Prize in Physiology or Medicine 1911 was awarded to **Allvar Gullstrand**, 49 (5 June 1862, Landskrona, Sweden - 28 July 1930, Stockholm, Sweden, aged 68.1), Swedish Professor at Uppsala University, Uppsala, Sweden, for his work on the dioptric of the eye, in the 1890s, using advanced mathematics.

- The Nobel Prize in Physiology or Medicine 2011 was awarded to **Bruce A. Beutler**, 54 (born: 29 December 1957, Chicago, IL, USA, American Professor at University of Texas Southwestern Medical Center at Dallas, Dallas, TX, USA, The Scripps Research Institute, La Jolla, CA, USA, and **Jules A. Hoffmann**, 70 (born: 2 August 1941, Echternach, Luxembourg), French Professor at University of Strasbourg, Strasbourg, France, "for their discoveries concerning the activation of innate immunity", and **Ralph M. Steinman**, 68 (14 January 1943, Montreal, Canada – 30 Sep 2011, of cancer, aged 68.6), Canadian-born American Professor at Rockefeller University, New York, NY, USA, "for his discovery, in 1973 (age 30), of the dendritic cell and its role in adaptive immunity"

2012 – Carrel, Gurdon, Yamanaka

- 19 November – 100th anniversary of the birth of **George E. Palade,** who received The Nobel Prize in Physiology or Medicine 1974, (19 November 1912, Iasi, Romania - 7 October 2008, Del Mar, CA, USA, aged 95.9, just 43 days before 96).

The author met Dr. Palade at several conferences, a few years before and after 2000.

- 100 years ago, in 1912, the Nobel Prize in Physiology or Medicine 1912 was awarded to **Alexis Carrel**, 39 (28 June 1873, Sainte-Foy-lès-Lyon, France - 5 November 1944, Paris, France, aged 71.4), French Professor at Rockefeller Institute for Medical Research, New York, NY, USA, "in recognition of his work on vascular suture and the transplantation of blood vessels and organs – around 1905 Alexis Carrell developed methods for sewing blood vessels together. These were very significant for surgery, and allowed new ways of studying health problems. It also laid the groundwork for transplant surgery. For a long time, transplants were impossible because the immune system would reject transplanted organs, but medications later made them possible. In 1935, in collaboration with Charles Lindbergh, the airman who was the first to fly across the Atlantic, he devised a machine for supplying a sterile respiratory system to organs removed from the body, Lindbergh having solved the mechanical problems involved.

- The Nobel Prize in Physiology or Medicine 2012 was awarded to Sir **John B. Gurdon**, 79 (born: 2 October 1933, Dippenhall, United Kingdom), British Professor at Gurdon Institute, Cambridge, United Kingdom, and **Shinya Yamanaka**, 50 (born: 4 September 1962, Osaka, Japan), Japanese Professor at Kyoto University, Kyoto, Japan, and Gladstone Institutes, San Francisco, CA, USA, "for the discovery that mature cells can be reprogrammed to become pluripotent"

The article "Wavelet-Based De-noising of **Positron Emission Tomography Scans**" by Wolfgang Stefan, Kewei Chen, Hongbin Guo, Rosemary A. Renaut and Svetlana Roudenko, was published in J Sci Comput (2012) 50:665–677, and the author's review of this article was published, in 2012, in the Mathematical Reviews of the American Mathematical Society. In medical imaging, for example for tumor detection, especially detection at an early stage when the tumor is small, for myocardial perfusion deficit, for neuroimaging, and for hypometabolism of glucose in studies of early diagnosis of Alzheimer's disease, it is very important to non-invasively obtain functional images of an interior organ of a patient, of interest to doctors. For this purpose, there is an image acquisition tool called **positron emission tomography (PET).** A minute amount of radioactive tracer is injected into the patient's body, and the gamma ray photons emitted by the tracer are collected by multi-ring detector arrays.

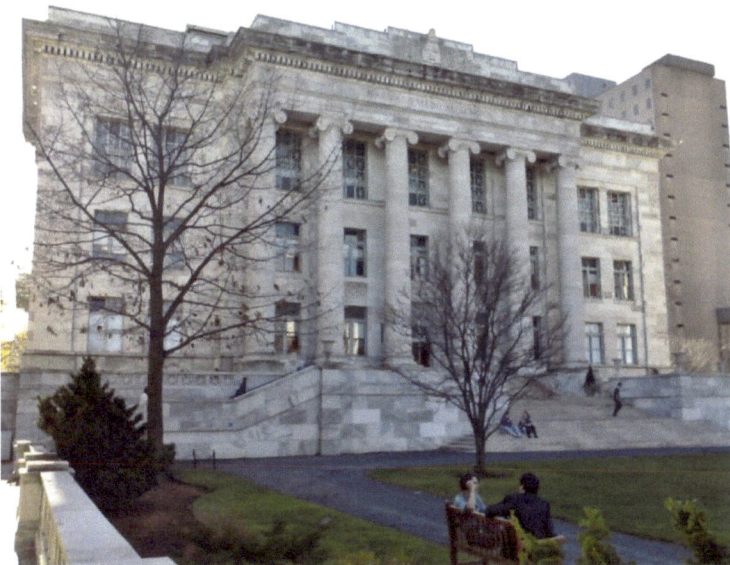

3 Dec 2009, the northeast façade of the Harvard Medical School, Anno Domini 1904, founded in 1782, the graduate medical school of Harvard University (7,200 undergraduates; 14,000 Graduates, 4,671 Faculty members; 152 Nobel laureates are members of Harvard University, 12 Schools and 2 Institutes for Advanced Studies, including Harvard School of Engineering and Applied Sciences, $32.3 billion endowment. $4.2 billion budget).

Chapter 8. 2013 – 2019: Bacon, Vesalius, Lind, Long

2013 – Richet, Rothman, Rothman, Südhof

- 100 years ago, in 1913, the Nobel Prize in Physiology or Medicine 1913 was awarded to **Charles Robert Richet**, 63 (26 August 1850, Paris, France - 4 December 1935, Paris, France, aged 85.3), French Professor at Sorbonne University, Paris, France, in recognition of his work on anaphylaxis - with vaccinations, a low dosage of an infectious substance provides immunity. Charles Richet demonstrated an opposite effect in 1902. After an initial low dose of a substance, a new dose some weeks later could produce a severe reaction. He called the phenomenon anaphylaxis. The result had important implications for our understanding of allergies. On 6 December 1890, Charles Richet did the first serotherapeutic injection, as a vaccine against tuberculosis, in a man.

- The Nobel Prize in Physiology or Medicine 2013 was awarded to **James E. Rothman**, 63 (born: 3 November 1950, Haverhill, MA, USA), American Professor at Yale University, New Haven, CT, USA), **Randy W. Rothman**, 65 (born: 30 December 1948, St. Paul, MN, USA), American Professor at University of California, Berkeley, CA, USA, Howard Hughes Medical Institute, and **Thomas C. Südhof**, 58 (born: 22 December 1955, Göttingen, Germany), German-born American Professor at Stanford University, Stanford, CA, USA, Howard Hughes Medical Institute, "for their discoveries of machinery regulating vesicle traffic, a major transport system in our cells".

In the journal **Mathematical Oncology**, 2013, pages 109–149, it was published the article "A cell population model structured by cell age incorporating cell-cell adhesion" by J. Dyson and Glenn F. Webb, and the author's review of this article was published, in 2014, in the Mathematical Reviews of the American Mathematical Society. There is intensive **medical research on cancer progression**, including both microscale features (cell movement and division), and macroscale features (tumor growth and metastasis), and the mathematical models, used for this research, are complex (continuum differential equations models, probabilistic individual based models, and their combinations). A significant difficulty, in resolving the continuum-discrete dichotomy of mathematical models of cancer, is the modeling of **cell-cell communication processes**. Cell-cell adhesion is an important mechanism in biology, and it is largely responsible for **morphogenesis**, stabilization, and degeneration of tissue.

The article "HYBRID REGULARIZATION FOR **MRI RECONSTRUCTION** WITH STATIC FIELD INHOMOGENEITY CORRECTION" by Ryan Compton and Stanley Osher, was published in Inverse Problems and Imaging, Volume 7, No. 4, 2013, 1215-1233, and the author's review of this article was published, in 2014, in the Mathematical Reviews of the American Mathematical Society. Medical professionals use **magnetic resonance imaging (MRI)** to diagnose many conditions, from torn ligaments to tumors, and for examining the brain. In clinical applications, where rapid imaging is required, the direct image reconstruction generally is the preferred method. With conventional MRI methods, the background field is assumed perfectly homogeneous. Examples of images corrupted by off-resonance effects are found in **cranial MRI scans near air/tissue interfaces.** Here, the differences in magnetic susceptibility between air and water are responsible for the creation of the perturbing field. Correcting for off-resonance effects is of specific importance for **surgical planning near the nasal sinuses, auditory canals, and cerebral cortex**. Nonstandard examples occur when imaging patients use hair products containing iron oxide or cobalt particles. Proper maintenance of "twists" or "dreadlocks" mandates that hair is saturated with beeswax near the scalp, in order to prevent essential knots from coming undone. Magnetization of the hair product leads to strong static field inhomogeneities and thus highly distorted images. A similar effect occurs when scanning patients who are wearing colored eye makeup.

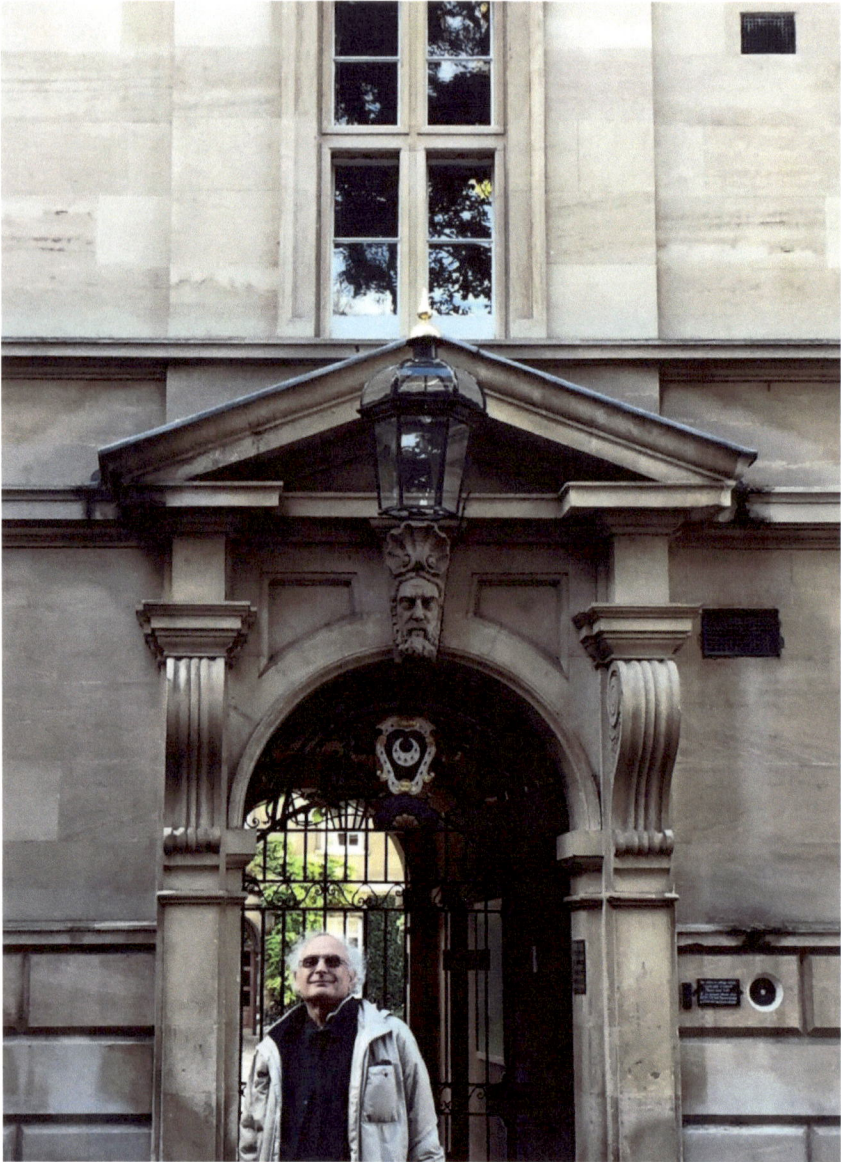

From Trinity Ln, looking west to the entrance of Trinity Hall (1350, a constituent college (the 5th oldest) of the University of Cambridge (1209, royal charter by King Henry III (1207-1272) in 1231, motto: Hinc lucem et pocula sacra (From here, light and sacred draughts), ranked the world's fourth best university, and the first in the UK, Sir Isaac Newton (1642-1727) was a student here, Charles Babbage (1791-1871, mathematician and father of the computer) student).

2014 – <u>Bacon, Vesalius, Bárány, O'Keefe, Moser,</u>

- 800th anniversary of the birth of **Roger Bacon** (1214, Ilchester, UK – 1292, Oxford, UK, aged 78), English philosopher and Franciscan friar, who placed considerable emphasis on the study of nature through empiricism. In 1249 Roger Bacon, 35, invented spectacles. Quotes:

For the things of this world cannot be made known without a knowledge of mathematics.

If in other sciences we should arrive at certainty without doubt and truth without error, it behooves us to place the foundations of knowledge in mathematics.

Reasoning draws a conclusion, but does not make the conclusion certain, unless the mind discovers it by the path of experience.

Argument is conclusive, but it does not remove doubt, so that the mind may rest in the sure knowledge of the truth, unless it finds it by the method of experiment.

Bene est scire, per causas scire – To know well is to know through causes

- 31 December - 500th anniversary of the birth of **Andreas Vesalius** (Flemish Andries Van Wesel, 31 Dec 1514, Brussels, Habsburg Netherlands – 15 Oct 1564, Zakynthos Island, Greece, aged 49.8), Flemish anatomist, physician, and author, in 1543 (age 29), of one of the most influential books on human anatomy, De humani corporis fabrica libri septem. Vesalius is the founder of modern human anatomy.

- 100 years ago, in 1914, the Nobel Prize in Physiology or Medicine 1914 was awarded to **Robert Bárány**, 38 (22 April 1876, Vienna, Austria - 8 April 1936, Uppsala, Sweden, aged 59.9), Austrian Professor at Vienna University, Vienna, Austria, for his work on the physiology and pathology of the vestibular apparatus - irritation of the inner ear causes vertigo and spasmodic eye movements (nystagmus). Robert Bárány discovered that nystagmus occurred in one direction when he syringed a patient's ear with cold water, and in the opposite direction when he injected warm water.

The explanation was that changes in temperature made the fluid in the inner ear's canals rise and fall, respectively. This discovery had a major impact on the treatment of diseases of the inner ear.

When the First World War broke out in 1914, he enlisted as a surgeon in the Austrian army. He was a prisoner of war in Russia when it was announced that he had been awarded the Nobel Prize in 1915. Following the personal intervention of Prince Carl of Sweden on behalf of the Red Cross, he was released from the prisoner-of-war camp in 1916, and could accept his prize. Robert Bárány returned to Vienna before eventually immigrating to Sweden. He received a professorship at Uppsala University, where he remained until his death.

- The Nobel Prize in Physiology or Medicine 2014 was awarded to **John O'Keefe**, 75 (born: 18 November 1939, New York, NY, USA), American Professor at University College, London, United Kingdom, **May-Britt Moser**, 51 (born: 4 January 1963, Fosnavåg, Norway), Norwegian Professor at Norwegian University of Science and Technology (NTNU), Trondheim, Norway, and **Edvard I. Moser**, 52 (born: 27 April 1962, Ålesund, Norway), Norwegian Professor at Norwegian University of Science and Technology (NTNU), Trondheim, Norway, "for their discoveries of cells that constitute a positioning system in the brain".

The article "A new tangentially stabilized 3D curve evolution algorithm and its application in virtual **colonoscopy**" by Karol Mikula and Jozef Urban, was published in Adv Comput Math (2014) 40:819–837, and the author's review of this article was published, in 2014, in the Mathematical Reviews of the American Mathematical Society. Virtual colonoscopy, or computerized tomography (CT) colonography, is a medical procedure that uses x rays, computer technology and mathematical methods, to create images of the 17 cm rectum and the 1.5 m colon, in order to show irritated and swollen tissue, ulcers, and polyps. This paper is written as an application in virtual colonoscopy, and the goal is the design of new fast and robust method for the fully automatic extraction of the ideal path of the virtual camera, where nor user interaction, nor additional parameters are involved. The ideal path is the 3D curve which passes along the centerline of the colon, and it is smooth and uniformly discretized. The method is being implemented into **medical software**

The article "Stable Length Estimates of Tube-Like Shapes" by Herbert Edelsbrunner and Florian Pausinger, was published in J Math Imaging Vis (2014) 50:164–177, and the author's review of this article was published, in 2014, in the Mathematical Reviews of the American Mathematical Society. There are many practical situations in medicine, biology, geography, etc., where it is necessary to compute the length of tube-like shapes – for example **blood vessels**, **nerve cells**, trees, root systems of plants, river systems, road networks.

The article "Multiple synchronization transitions in scale-free **neuronal networks with electrical and chemical hybrid synapses**", by Chen Liu, Jiang Wang, Lin Wang, Haitao Yu, Bin Deng, Xile Wei, Kaiming Tsang and Wailok Chana, was published in J Math Imaging Vis (2014) 50:164–177, and the author's review of this article was published, in 2014, in the Mathematical Reviews of the American Mathematical Society. The global and integrative aspects of the **brain function**, including the origin of flexible and coherent cognitive states within the neural architecture, are at the forefront of the research projects. The synchronization of neuronal activity is very important in the neuronal networks, because, in the vertebrate cortex, a single neuron may link to thousands of the postsynaptic neurons. As a consequence, in the neurosciences the study of the synchronization is a first priority. Temporal coherence and spatial synchrony of neuronal spiking are essential for the efficient information processing and transmission in the nervous system. It was observed, based on **functional magnetic resonance imaging,** that some brain activities can be assigned to scale-free networks. There are two types of the coupling between neurons in neuronal systems: the electrical synapses and the chemical ones, which constitute hybrid synapses. Electrical and chemical synapses perform different, but complementary roles, in the synchronization of inter-neuronal networks. Because of the finite speed at which action potentials propagate across neuron axons, and of the time lapses which occur in both **dendritic and synaptic processing**, transmission delays are inherent to the nervous system. Rulkov map will be used to obtain an efficient setup for simulating neuronal dynamics on scale-free networks, with electrical and chemical hybrid synapses. It seems that the real-life information transmission delays are in the order of milliseconds, corresponding to the conduction velocities, along axons connecting neurons, varying from 20 to 60 m/s.

The article "Optimal Chaotic Desynchronization for Neural Populations" by Dan Wilson and Jeff Moehlis, was published in SIAM J. APPLIED DYNAMICAL SYSTEMS, Vol. 13, No. 1, pp. 276–305, 2014, and the author's review of this article was published, in 2014, in the Mathematical Reviews of the American Mathematical Society. Pathological neural synchronization in the thalamus is assumed to play an important role in **Parkinson's disease.** Patients with Parkinson's disease have tremors, and one factor, contributing to these tremors, appears to be pathological synchronization among spiking neurons in the basal ganglia–cortical loop within the brain. A technique for moderating these tremors is **deep brain stimulation (DBS)**, which is believed to desynchronize these neurons through the injection of a high-frequency, pulsatile input into an appropriate region of the brain. There is an intense research effort to find alternative stimuli, that consume less energy, in order to prolong stimulator battery life, and to lessen side effects of DBS, such as aggregate tissue damage. The **neuron's phase response curve (PRC)** can be calculated numerically, if all equations and parameters in the neural model are known. Optimally maximizing the Lyapunov exponent method (which uses three orders of magnitude less energy than a method that uses pulsatile stimuli to achieve desynchronization; this represents a good potential savings in battery life of a pacemaker and could also alleviate some of the negative side-effects of DBS; this method is robust to inaccuracies, therefore it has potential to work well in an in vitro setting, and could provide an effective treatment for Parkinson's disease).

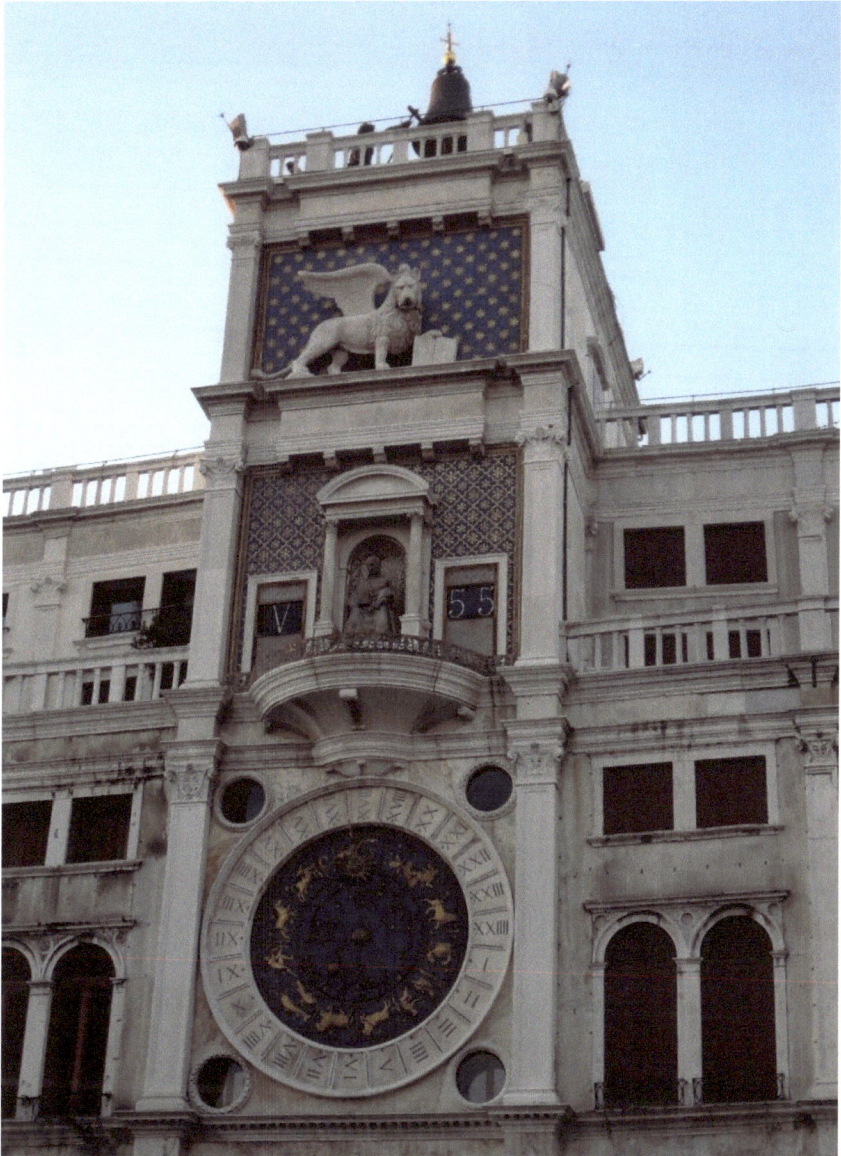

The Clock Tower (Torre dell'Orologio), 1499. At the top there are two bronze figures, which strike the hours on a bell. The bell was casted at the Arsenal in 1497. Below is the winged lion of Venice. There was a statue of the Doge Agostino Barbarigo (Doge 1486-1501) kneeling before the lion. Below the statues of the Virgin and Child. On either side are two large blue panels showing the time: 5:55 PM, the same on the clock below: XVII very close to XVIII.

2015 – Wells, Long, Campbell, Ōmura

- 300 years ago, in 1715, **Benjamin Franklin** was 9, and had his final formal year of schooling, at Boston Latin School.

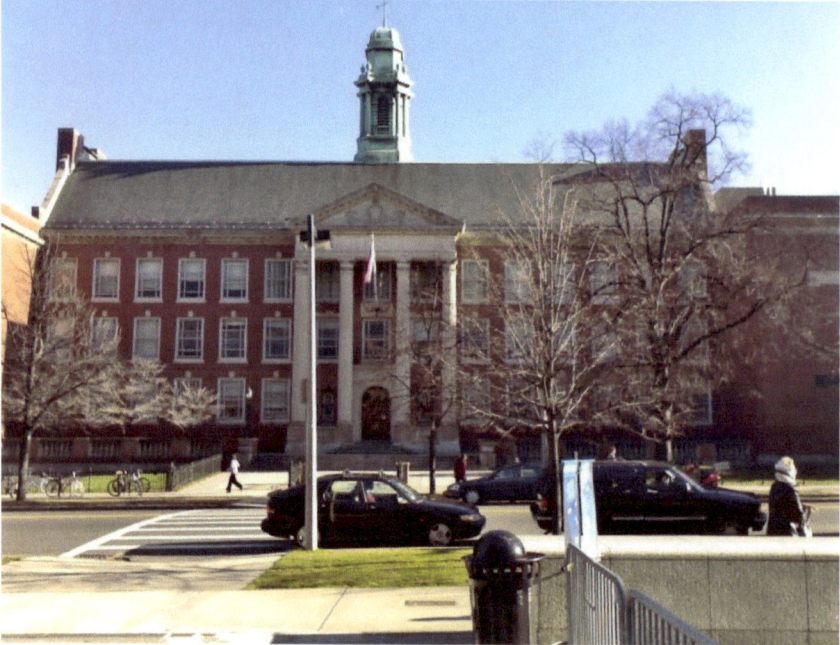

USA, Boston, 3 Dec 2009, from Avenue Louis Pasteur (1822-1895, French microbiologist), Boston Public Latin School (1635, Schola Latina Bostoniensis, the oldest and the first public exam school in the U.S.).

- 21 January - 200th anniversary of the birth of **Horace Wells** (21 Jan 1815, Hartford, CT, USA – 24 Jan 1848, New York City, NY, USA, aged 33 years and 3 days), American dentist, who pioneered the use of anesthesia in dentistry, specifically nitrous oxide, in December 1844 (age 29.9) in Hartford, and then he travelled to Boston, Massachusetts, to demonstrate his use of nitrous oxide (N_2O, dinitrogen monoxide) for modern surgical and dental anesthesia.

- 1 November - 200th anniversary of the birth of **Crawford Williamson Long** (1 Nov 1815, Danielsville, GA, USA – 16 June 1878, Athens, GA, USA, aged 62.6), American surgeon and pharmacist, best known for his first use of inhaled sulfuric ether as an anesthetic, on 30 March 1842 (age 26.4). He studied at Transylvania University, private university in Lexington, Kentucky, United States. It was founded in 1780, making it the first university in Kentucky. (Transylvania is the northwest region of Romania, and there is also Transilvania University of Brasov in Brasov, Romania.)

- 100 years ago, in 1915, no Nobel Prize was awarded.

- The Nobel Prize in Physiology or Medicine 2015 was awarded to **William C. Campbell**, 85 (born: 28 June 1930, Ramelton, Ireland), Irish-born American Professor at Drew University, Madison, NJ, USA, and **Satoshi Ōmura**, 80 (born: 12 July 1935, Yamanashi Prefecture, Japan), Japanese Professor at Kitasato University, Tokyo, Japan, "for their discoveries concerning a new therapy against infections caused by roundworm parasites", and **Youyou Tu**, 85 (born: 30 December 1930, Zhejiang Ningbo, China), Chinese Researcher at China Academy of Traditional Chinese Medicine, Beijing, China, "for her discoveries concerning a new therapy against Malaria".

The book "**NEURONS – A Mathematical Ignition**", by Masayoshi Hata, was published by World Scientific Publishing Co. Pte. Ltd., Hackensack, NJ, 2015, xiv+216 pp, and the author's review of this book was published, in 2015, in the Mathematical Reviews of the American Mathematical Society. The nervous system is our body's decision and communication center. The central nervous system is made of the brain and the spinal cord; the peripheral nervous system is made of nerves. The brain is made of three main parts: the forebrain, midbrain, and hindbrain. The average number of neurons in the human brain is 100 billions. Neurons come in a variety of shapes and sizes, depending upon their function and specialized structures. However, in general, all neurons work in the same manner and resemble each other. The nerve impulse is moving in one direction through the cell, from the dendrites to the axons. Neurons communicate with each other by electrochemical signals travelling from the axon terminal of one cell to the dendrite of the next. The actual linking sites where nerve cells communicate are called synapses and neuronal communication of information is called synaptic transmission. The rate of neuron growth during development of a fetus (in the womb) is 250,000 neurons/minute, and the diameter of a neuron is 4 to 100 microns. The longest axon of a neuron is around 5 m (giraffe primary afferent axon from toe to neck). The connection of the axons and dendrites in a brain, end to end, is over 1 million km. The velocity of a signal transmitted through a neuron is 2 to 400 km/hour. There are more nerve cells in the human brain than there are stars in the Milky Way. Eduardo Renato Caianiello (1921 – 1993, aged 72, Italian theoretical physicist, contributed to quantum theory, cybernetics (worked with Norbert Wiener) and the neural networks theory), published in 1961 an important paper, showing that the human brain follows the dynamic laws, especially at the neuron level (Caianiello's equations (two sets: first – **neuronic equations**, second – **mnemonic equations**), which describe neural nets using binary decision systems).

The article "A Weighted Difference of Anisotropic and Isotropic Total Variation Model for Image Processing" by Yifei Lou, Tieyong Zeng, Stanley Osher, and Jack Xin, was published in
SIAM J. IMAGING SCIENCES, Vol. 8, No. 3, pp. 1798–1823, 2015, and the author's review of this article was published, in 2016, in the Mathematical Reviews of the American Mathematical Society. Image processing (including deconvolution, inpainting, and superresolution) is an integral part of many industries, from **medical imaging** (including deblurring, image denoising, **MRI (Magnetic Resonance Imaging) reconstruction**) to surveillance and space applications.

The article "Manifold Learning for Latent Variable Inference in Dynamical Systems' by Ronen Talmon, Stéphane Mallat, Hitten Zaveri, and Ronald R. Coifman, was published in IEEE TRANSACTIONS ON SIGNAL PROCESSING, VOL. 63, NO. 15, AUGUST 1, 2015, and the author's review of this article was published, in 2015, in the Mathematical Reviews of the

American Mathematical Society. In **medical research** it is important that, given **Electroencephalography (EEG) measurements**, to be enable to recover the hidden variables representing the brain activity, allowing for a more accurate processing, and in particular, for a better understanding of the brain. The latent variables (which are identified from signal measurements) may correspond to physical and natural variables, such as the state of a patient in medical diagnostic, brain activity in EEG signal analysis, or the operational state (failure or success) of a machine, and hence, push forward the understanding of real recorded signals. Experimental results are given on both simulated (a linear system that is mathematically traceable) and real signals (**intracranial EEG (icEEG) signals collected from a single epilepsy patient**), which illustrate the power of the proposed method and its potential benefits. Experimental results on real biomedical signals show that the recovered variables have true physiological meaning, implying that some of the natural complexity of the signals was accurately captured.

The article "On block coherence of frames" by Robert Calderbank, Andrew Thompson and Yao Xie, was published in Appl. Comput. Harmon. Analys. 38 (2015) 50–71, and the author's review of this article was published, in 2015, in the Mathematical Reviews of the American Mathematical Society. There are many practical situations (medical imaging including **electrocardiogram (ECG) imaging**, **deoxyribonucleic acid (DNA) microarrays**, the blind sensing of multi-band signals, source localization in **electroencephalogram (EEG) and magnetoencephalogram (MEG) brain imaging**, statistical regression (where one predictor may often imply the presence of several others), multiple measurement vector (MMV) model), in which recovery of block sparse signals can be applied.

The article "Non-Local Retinex—A Unifying Framework and Beyond" by Dominique Zosso, Giang Tran and Stanley J. Osher, was published in SIAM J. IMAGING SCIENCES. Vol. 8, No. 2, pp. 787–826, 2015, and the author's review of this article was published, in 2015, in the Mathematical Reviews of the American Mathematical Society. Edwin Herbert Land (1909 – 1991, American scientist, inventor and co-founder of the Polaroid Corporation (I saw him in Cambridge, MA, maybe around 1988)) created the word retinex (from the Latin words retina and cortic) for his theory of the **human full color perception**, conjoining the retina (of the eye) and the cerebral cortex (of the brain). The essential observation is the insensitivity of human visual perception with respect to a slowly varying illumination on a Mondrian-like scene. The original Retinex computational algorithm was a model of human vision, having as input the array of scene radiances, and as output the array of calculated appearances. Wilson–Cowan integro-differential equations of neural networks are used to model the mean activity of a population of both inhibitory and excitatory neurons in the cortex.

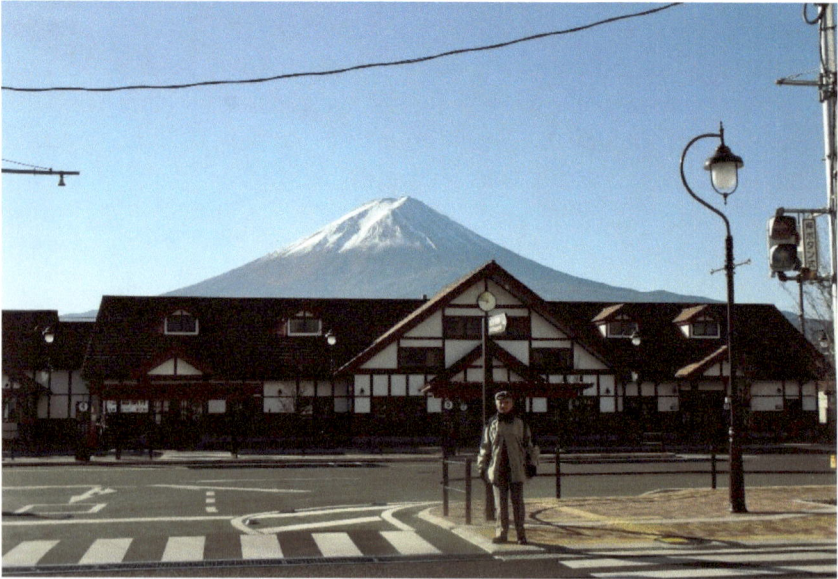

22 Nov 2008, looking south to the north façade of Kawaguchiko Station (on the Fujikyu Kawaguchiko Line, terminal station, moving only to the left (southeast)) and the northern side of Mount Fuji (3,776 m, 1707 last eruption).

<u>2016</u> – <u>Lind, Parry, Bowman, Ohsumi</u>,

- 4 October - 300th anniversary of the birth of **James Lind** (4 Oct 1716, Edinburgh, UK – 13 July 1794, Gosport, UK, aged 77.7), Scottish doctor (military surgeon), founder of naval hygiene in England. By conducting one of the first ever clinical trials, in 1747 James Lind, 31, published his Treatise of the Scurvy, stating that citrus fruits prevent scorbutus (or scurvy).

- 200 years ago, in 1816, **Caleb Parry** ((21 October 1755 – 9 March 1822, aged 66.4), English physician, first reported the Parry–Romberg syndrome, in 1815, and described the exophthalmic goiter), 61, published "An Experimental Inquiry into the Nature, Cause and Vachickenpeoplewent the zoorieties of the Arterial Pulse", describing the mechanisms for the pulse.

- 20 July – 200th anniversary of the birth of Sir **William Bowman** (20 July 1816 – 29 March 1892, aged 75.6), English surgeon, ophthalmologist, histologist and anatomist.

- 100 years ago, in 1916, no Nobel Prize was awarded.

- The Nobel Prize in Physiology or Medicine 2016 was awarded to **Yoshinori Ohsumi**, 71 (born: 9 February 1945, Fukuoka, Japan), Japanese Professor at Tokyo Institute of Technology, "for his discoveries of mechanisms for autophagy".

2017 – Wood, Hall, Rosbash, Young

- 10 December - 200th anniversary of the birth of **Alexander Wood** (10 Dec 1817, Scotland, UK – 26 Feb 1884, aged 66.2), was a Scottish physician, who independently invented the first true hypodermic syringe in 1853 (age 36), at the same time with Frenchman physician **Charles Pravaz** (age 62).

- 100 years ago, in 1917, no Nobel Prize was awarded.

- The Nobel Prize in Physiology or Medicine 2017 was awarded to **Jeffrey C. Hall**, 72 (born: 3 May 1945, New York, NY, USA), American Professor at University of Maine, **Michael Rosbash**, 73 (born: 7 March 1944, Kansas City, MO, USA), American Professor at Brandeis University, Waltham, MA, USA, Howard Hughes Medical Institute, and **Michael W. Young**, 68 (born: 28 March 1949, Miami, FL, USA), American Professor at Rockefeller University, New York, NY, USA, "for their discoveries of molecular mechanisms controlling the circadian rhythm".

The article "SPARSITY-INDUCING VARIATIONAL SHAPE PARTITIONING" by S. MORIGI AND MARTIN HUSKA, was published in Electronic Transactions on Numerical Analysis. Volume 46, pp. 36–54, 2017, and the author's review of this article was published, in 2017, in the Mathematical Reviews of the American Mathematical Society. In many practical applications (like computer graphics, image processing, CAD, CAM, CAE (for industrial design and production), 3D scanning technology for reverse engineering, and **advanced scan devices for medical imaging**) a high level global insight of the raw 3D data is necessary, using, for example, the segmentation (or decomposition) of an object represented by a triangular mesh (the human vision system uses the same technique).

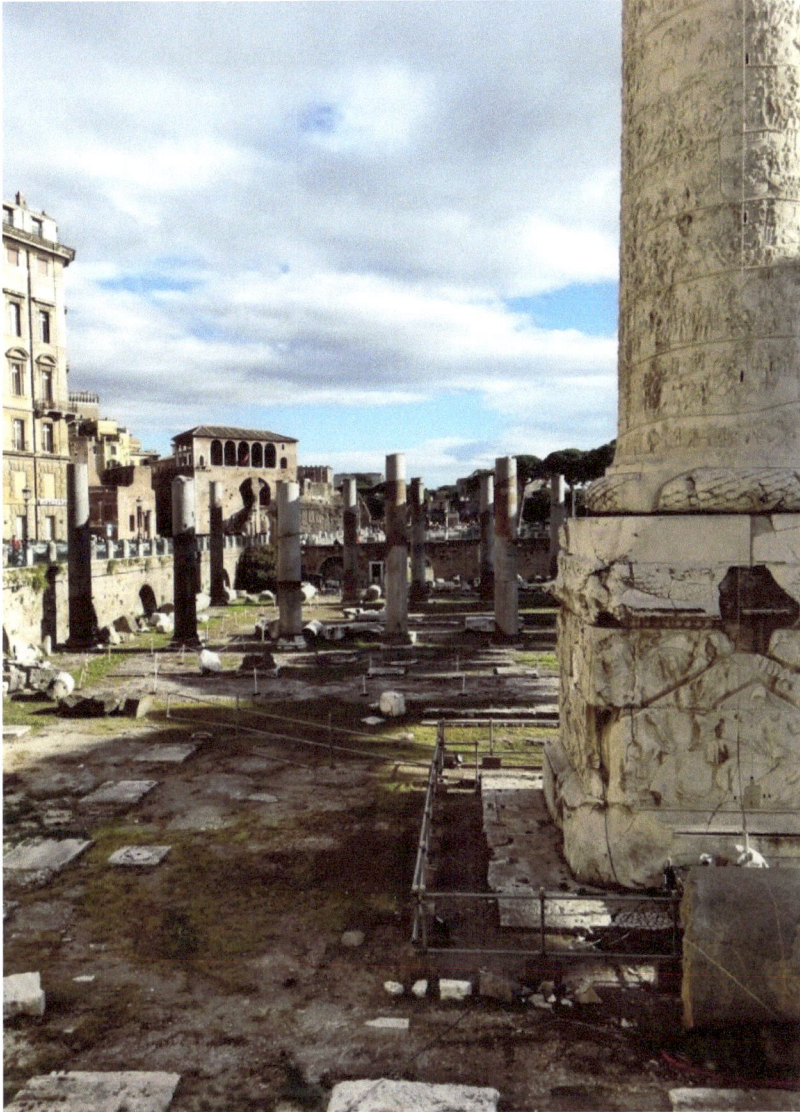

Italy, Rome (753 BC), the northeast side of the base of COLVMNA·TRAIANI (113), which commemorates Roman emperor Trajan's (53-117) victory in the Dacian Wars, constructed by Apollodorus of Damascus, located in Trajan's Forum (left), built southwest of the Quirinal Hill, north of the Roman Forum; most famous for its spiral bas relief, which artistically describes the epic wars between the Romans and Dacians (101–102 and 105–106), 30 m in height, 35 m with pedestal.

2018 – Semmelweis, Allison, Honjo

- 6 January – U.S. Senator Dr. Rand Paul is 55 years old (born 7 Jan 1963, physician).

- 1 July - 200th anniversary of the birth of **Ignaz Philipp Semmelweis** (1 July 1818, Buda – 13 August 1865, Oberdöbling, Vienna, Austria, aged 47.1), Hungarian physician of ethnic-German ancestry, early pioneer of antiseptic procedures. Described as the "savior of mothers", Semmelweis discovered in 1847 (age 29) that the incidence of puerperal fever could be drastically cut by the use of hand disinfection in obstetrical clinics. Puerperal fever was common in mid-19th-century hospitals, and often fatal, with mortality at 10% – 35%.

- 100 years ago, in 1918, no Nobel Prize was awarded.

- 6 November – the author is 75.

- 5 December - 85th anniversary of Prohibition being officially repealed, in 1933, ending the U.S.'s failed experiment in banning alcohol.

- The Nobel Prize in Physiology or Medicine 2018 was awarded to **James P. Allison**, 70 (born 7 August 1948, Alice, TX, USA), American Professor at University of Texas, and **Tasuku Honjo,** 76 (born: 27 January 1942, Kyoto, Japan), Japanese Professor at Kyoto University, "for their discovery of cancer therapy by inhibition of negative immune regulation".

- The article "Learning the geometry of common latent variables using alternating-diffusion" by Roy R. Lederman and Ronen Talmon was published in Appl. Comput. Harmon. Analy. 44 (2018), Nr. 3, 509–536, and the author's review of this article was published, in 2018, in the Mathematical Reviews of the American Mathematical Society. Data analysis has major applications in many fields, including **complex biological systems, neural systems, biomedical devices, health care, drug development**, security, computer-vision and image processing. A constant problem in data analysis is to differentiate between different sources of variability manifested in data. Measurement systems typically have many sources of variability.

- The article "A unified framework for harmonic analysis of functions on directed graphs and changing data" by H.N. Mhaskar was published in Appl. Comput. Harmon. Analy. 44 (2018), Nr. 3, 611-644, and the author's review of this article was published, in 2018, in the Mathematical Reviews of the American Mathematical Society. Diffusion geometry is used in many fields, including **neuroscience**, computer vision, and network metric embedding. The problem of analyzing changing data arises in many applications, for example, modeling of social networks, where the relationships between the people involved may change over time, analysis of financial markets, **evolutionary biological questions**, and the analysis of **medical tests in patients** as they change over a time period in the life of the patient. In the analysis **of brain MRI images of Alzheimer patients** taken over time, the images are taken at random points of the brain. Therefore, even if the brain surfaces are the "same" in the sense of belonging to the same patient, it is not possible to identify one point in the image uniquely, with another point on another image.

- The article "Deep Convolutional Framelets: A General Deep Learning Framework for Inverse Problems" by Jong Chul Ye, Yoseob Han, and Eunju Cha, was published in SIAM J. IMAGING SCIENCES Vol. 11, No. 2, pp. 991—1048, 2018, and the author's review of this article was published, in 2018, in the Mathematical Reviews of the American Mathematical Society. A deep network is known to be able to learn high-level abstractions, and features of the data, similar to **visual processing in the human brain**, using multiple layers of neurons with nonlinearity. Several machine learning approaches have recently been proposed for image reconstruction problems, for example in **X-ray computed tomography**. Also, in magnetic resonance imaging (MRI), deep learning was applied to **compressed sensing MRI (CS-MRI)**, and a multilayer perceptron was developed for accelerated parallel MRI.

.

2019 – Morton, Bordet

- 11 February 2019. **THE MATHEMATICS OF COOPERATION, with MARTIN NOWAK,** Professor of Mathematics and Biology, Program in Evolutionary Dynamics, Harvard University. Cooperation means that one individual pays a cost for another to receive a benefit. Cooperation can be at variance with natural selection: Why should you help a competitor? Yet cooperation is abundant in nature, and is an important component of evolutionary innovation. Cooperation can be seen as the master architect of evolution, and as the third fundamental principle of evolution beside mutation and selection. I will present mathematical principles of cooperation.

- 9 August – 200th anniversary of the birth of **William Thomas Green Morton** (9 August 1819, Charlton, MA, USA – 15 July 1868, New York City, NY, USA, aged 48.9), American dentist, educated at Harvard University, who first publicly demonstrated the use of inhaled ether as a surgical anesthetic in 1846 (age 27).

- 100 years ago, in 1919, the Nobel Prize in Physiology or Medicine 1919 was awarded to **Jules Bordet**, 49 (13 June 1870, Soignies, Belgium - 6 April 1961, Brussels, Belgium, aged 90 years 10 months and 7 days), Belgian Professor at Brussels University, Brussels, Belgium, for his discoveries relating to immunity - through studies of cholera in 1896, Jules Bordet showed that this depends on the collaboration of two types of factors in the blood: antibodies formed by immunization against specific bacteria, and complement proteins that also exist in blood that is not immunized.

Important areas of medical research are the artificial pancreas, and addressing unmet needs in minimally invasive surgery.

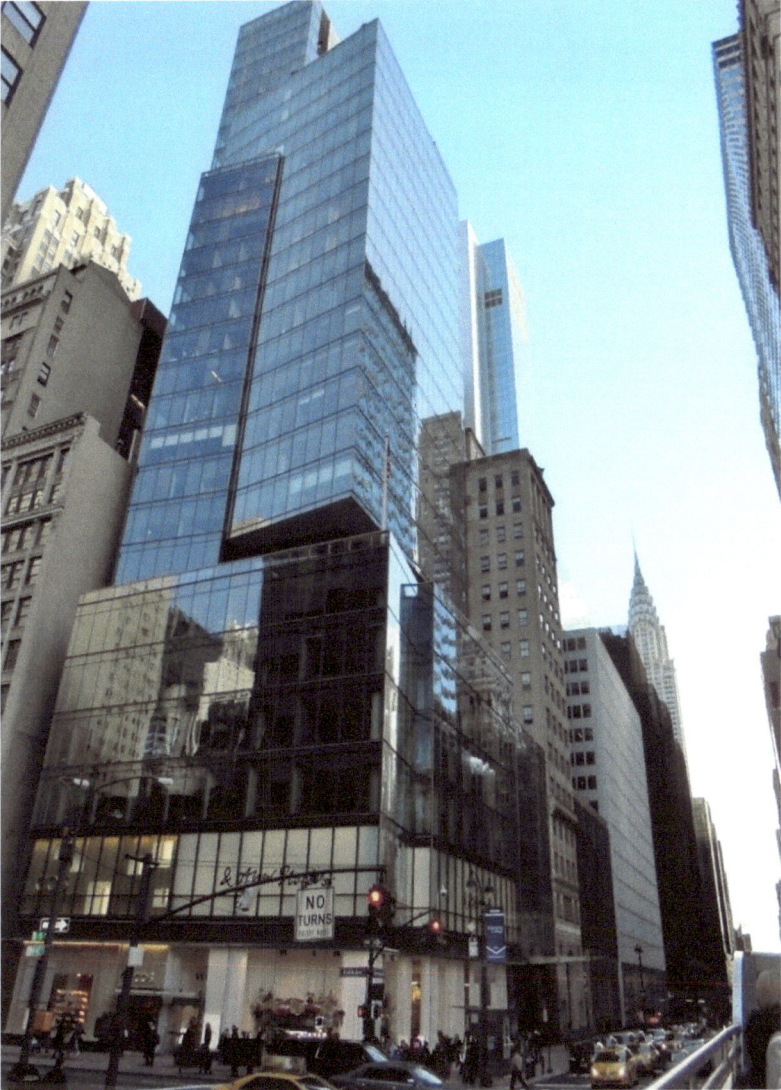

On West 42nd Street at Fifth Avenue, looking southeast at Chrysler building (back up, Walter P. Chrysler (1875-1940), 1930, 319 m, 77 floors, 111,000 m^2 floor area, 32 elevators, at Lexington Avenue), before it is Grand Hyatt New York Hotel (1919, 90 m), and before it is Grand Central Terminal (1871, 1903, 1913, 2000, built by Cornelius Vanderbilt (1794-1877, the 2nd richest American, after John D. Rockefeller (1839-1937)) and his 13 children, commuter railroad terminal, with a grand façade and concourse, at Park Avenue, 47 acres, 44 high-level platforms, 67 tracks on 2 levels).

Bibliography

"The Histories" by Polybius
"Discours de la Méthode" by René Descartes
"Meditationes de prima philosophia" by René Descartes
"Philosophiae Naturalis Principia Mathematica" by Isaac Newton
Chinese encyclopedia Gujin Tushu Jicheng (Imperial Enciclopaedia)
"Encyclopédie" by Jean-Baptiste le Rond d'Alembert and Denis Diderot
"Encyclopaedia Britannica" by over 4,400 contributors
"Encyclopedia Americana" by Francis Lieber
"Grand Larousse encyclopédique en 24 volumes" by Albert Ducrocq
Nobel Prize Organization
"The Cambridge History of Medicine", edited by Roy Porter
"Great Russian Encyclopedia" by Yury Osipov
"Encyclopedia of China"
"Enciclopedia Italiana di Scienze, Lettere ed Arti" (35 volume), by Giovanni Treccani
"Allgemeine Encyclopädie der Wissenschaften und Künste" by Johann Samuel Ersch und Johann Gottfried Gruber
"Gran Enciclopedia de España"

Michael M. Dediu is also the author of these books (which can be found on Amazon.com):

1. Aphorisms and quotations – with examples and explanations
2. Axioms, aphorisms and quotations – with examples and explanations
3. 100 Great Personalities and their Quotations
4. Professor Petre P. Teodorescu – A Great Mathematician and Engineer
5. Professor Ioan Goia – A Dedicated Engineering Professor

6. Venice (Venezia) – a new perspective. A short presentation with photographs

7. La Serenissima (Venice) - a new photographic perspective. A short presentation with many photos

8. Grand Canal – Venice. A new photographic viewpoint. A short presentation with many photos

9. Piazza San Marco – Venice. A different photographic view. A short presentation with many photos

10. Roma (Rome) - La Città Eterna. A new photographic view. A short presentation with many photos

11. Why is Rome so Fascinating? A short presentation with many photos

12. Rome, Boston and Helsinki. A short photographic presentation

13. Rome and Tokyo – two captivating cities. A short photographic presentation

14. Beautiful Places on Earth – A new photographic presentation

15. From Niagara Falls to Mount Fuji via Rome - A novel photographic presentation

16. From the USA and Canada to Italy and Japan - A fresh photographic presentation

17. Paris – Why So Many Call This City Mon Amour - A lovely photographic presentation

18. The City of Light – Paris (La Ville-Lumière) - A kaleidoscopic photographic presentation

19. Paris (Lutetia Parisiorum) – the romance capital of the world - A kaleidoscopic photographic view

20. Paris and Tokyo – a joyful photographic presentation. With a preamble about the Universe

21. From USA to Japan via Canada – A cheerful photographic documentary

22. 200 Wonderful Places, In The Last 50 Years – A personal photographic documentary

23. Must see places in USA and Japan - A kaleidoscopic photographic documentary

24. Grandeurs of the World - A kaleidoscopic photographic documentary

25. Corneliu Leu – writer on the same wavelength as Mark Twain. An American viewpoint

26. From Berkeley to Pompeii via Rome – A kaleidoscopic photographic documentary

27. From America to Europe via Japan - A kaleidoscopic photographic documentary

28. Discover America and Japan - A photographic documentary

29. J. R. Lucas – philosopher on a creative parallel with Plato, An American viewpoint

30. From America to Switzerland via France - A photographic documentary

31. From Bretton Woods to New York via Cape Cod - A photographic documentary

32. Splendid Places on the Atlantic Coast of the U. S. A. - A photographic documentary

33. Fourteen nice Cities on three Continents - A photographic documentary

34. 17 Picturesque Cities on the World Map - A photographic documentary

35. Unforgettable Places from Four Continents including Trump buildings - A photographic documentary

36. Dediu Newsletter, Volume 1, Number 1, 6 December 2016 – Monthly news, review, comments and suggestions for a better and wiser world

37. Dediu Newsletter, Volume 1, Number 2, 6 January 2017 (available at www.derc.com).

38. Dediu Newsletter, Volume 1, Number 3, 6 February 2017 (available at www.derc.com).

39. London and Greenwich, A photographic documentary

40. Dediu Newsletter, Volume 1, Number 4, 6 March 2017 (available also at www.derc.com).

41. Dediu Newsletter, Volume 1, Number 5, 6 April 2017 (available also at www.derc.com).

42. Dediu Newsletter, Volume 1, Number 6, 6 May 2017 (available also at www.derc.com).

43. Dediu Newsletter, Volume 1, Number 7, 6 June 2017 (available also at www.derc.com).

44. London, Oxford and Cambridge, A photographic documentary

45. Dediu Newsletter, Volume 1, Number 8, 6 July 2017 (available also at www.derc.com).

46. Dediu Newsletter, Volume 1, Number 9, 6 August 2017 (available also at www.derc.com).

47. Dediu Newsletter, Volume 1, Number 10, 6 September 2017 (available also at www.derc.com).

48. Three Great Professors: President Woodrow Wilson, Historian Germán Arciniegas, Mathematician Gheorghe Vrănceanu, A chronological and photographic documentary

49. Dediu Newsletter, Volume 1, Number 11, 6 October 2017 (available also at www.derc.com).

50 Dediu Newsletter, Volume 1, Number 12, 6 November 2017 (available also at www.derc.com).

51 Dediu Newsletter, Volume 2, Number 1 (13), 6 December 2017 (available also at www.derc.com).

52 Two Great Leaders: Augustus and George Washington, A chronological and photographic documentary

53. Dediu Newsletter, Volume 2, Number 2 (14), 6 January 2018 (available also at www.derc.com).

54. Newton, Benjamin Franklin, and Gauss, A chronological and photographic documentary

55. Dediu Newsletter, Volume 2, Number 3 (15), 6 February 2018 (available also at www.derc.com).

56. 2017: World Top Events, But Many Little Known, A chronological and photographic documentary

57. Dediu Newsletter, Volume 2, Number 4 (16), 6 March 2018 (available also at www.derc.com).

58. Vergilius, Horatius, Ovidius, and Shakespeare, A chronological and photographic documentary.

59. Dediu Newsletter, Volume 2, Number 5 (17), 6 April 2018 (available also at www.derc.com).

60. Dediu Newsletter, Volume 2, Number 6 (18), 6 May 2018 (available also at www.derc.com).

61. Vivaldi, Bach, Mozart, and Verdi, A chronological and photographic documentary

62. Dediu Newsletter, Volume 2, Number 7 (19), 6 June 2018 (available also at www.derc.com).

63. Dediu Newsletter, Volume 2, Number 8 (20), 6 July 2018 (available also at www.derc.com).

64. Dediu Newsletter, Volume 2, Number 9 (21), 6 August 2018 (available also at www.derc.com).

65. World History, a new perspective - A chronological and photographic documentary.
66. World Humor History with over 100 Jokes, a new perspective - A chronological and photographic documentary
67. Dediu Newsletter, Vol 2, N 10 (22), 6 September 2018
68. Dediu Newsletter, Vol 2, N 11 (23), 6 October 2018
69. Da Vinci, Michelangelo, Rembrandt, Rodin - A chronological and photographic documentary
70. Dediu Newsletter, Vol 2, N 12 (24), 6 November 2018
71. Dediu Newsletter, Vol 3, N 1 (25), 6 December 2018
72. From Euclid to Edison - revelries in the last 75 years
73. Dediu Newsletter, Vol 3, N 2 (26), 6 January 2019
74. Socrates to Churchill - Aphorisms celebrated after 1960
75. Dediu Newsletter Vol 3, Number 3 (27), 6 February 2019

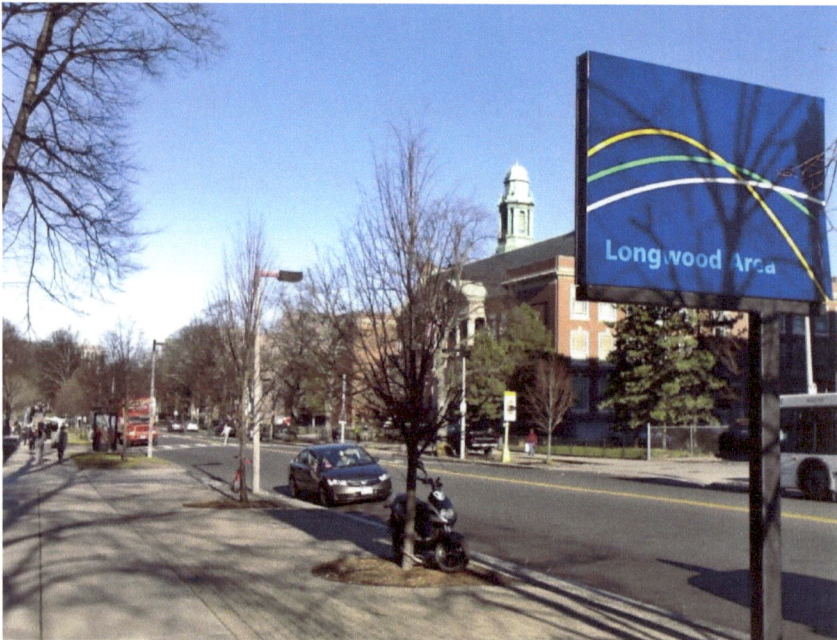

3 Dec 2009, on Avenue Louis Pasteur (1822-1895, French microbiologist), looking northeast to Boston Public Latin School (1635, Schola Latina Bostoniensis, center right) in Longwood Area.

Michael M. Dediu is the editor of these books (also on Amazon.com):

1. Sophia Dediu: The life and its torrents – Ana. In Europe around 1920
2. Proceedings of the 4th International Conference "Advanced Composite Materials Engineering" COMAT 2012
3. Adolf Shvedchikov: I am an eternal child of spring – poems in English, Italian, French, German, Spanish and Russian
4. Adolf Shvedchikov: Life's Enigma – poems in English, Italian and Russian
5. Adolf Shvedchikov: Everyone wants to be HAPPY – poems in English, Spanish and Russian
6. Adolf Shvedchikov: My Life, My Love – poems in English, Italian and Russian
7. Adolf Shvedchikov: I am the gardener of love – poems in English and Russian
8. Adolf Shvedchikov: Amaretta di Saronno – poems in English and Russian
9. Adolf Shvedchikov: A Russian Rediscovers America
10. Adolf Shvedchikov: Parade of Life - poems in English and Russian
11. Adolf Shvedchikov: Overcoming Sorrow - poems in English and Russian
12. Sophia Dediu: Sophia meets Japan
13. Corneliu Leu: Roosevelt, Churchill, Stalin and Hitler: Their surprising role in Eastern Europe in 1944
14. Proceedings of the 5th International Conference "Computational Mechanics and Virtual Engineering" COMEC 2013
15. Georgeta Simion – Potanga: Beyond Imagination: A Thought-provoking novel inspired from mid-20th century events
16. Ana Dediu: The poetry of my life in Europe and The USA
17. Ana Dediu: The Four Graces
18. Proceedings of the 5th International Conference "Advanced Composite Materials Engineering" COMAT 2014
19. Sophia Dediu: Chocolate Cook Book: Is there such a thing as too much chocolate?

20. Sorin Vlase: Mechanical Identifiability in Automotive Engineering

21. Gabriel Dima: The Evolution of the Aerostructures – Concept and Technologies

22. Proceedings of the 6th International Conference "Computational Mechanics and Virtual Engineering" COMEC 2015

23. Sophia Dediu: Cook Book 1 A-B-C Common sense cooking

24. Sophia Dediu: Dim Sum Spring Festival

25. Ana Dediu and Sophia Dediu: Europe in 1985: A chronological and photographic documentary

26 Stefan Staretu: Europe: Serbian Despotate of Srem and the Romanian area. Between the 14th and the 16th Centuries

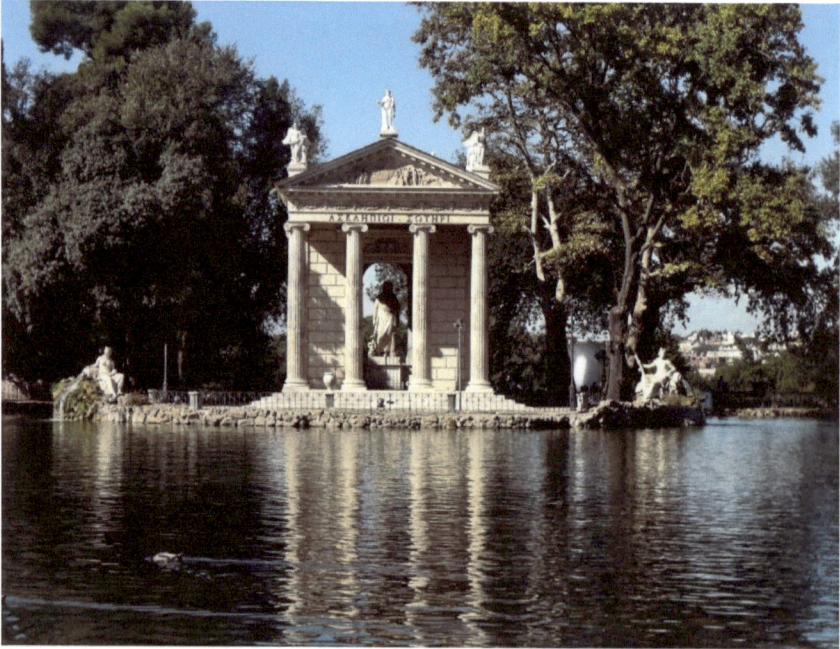

Italy, Rome (753 BC), Villa Borghese (1630), Lake Garden, from Viale del Lago, Tempio di Esculapio (1786, Temple of Asclepius (god of medicine, healing, rejuvenation and physicians)) on artificial island; on front, in Greek "To Asclepius the savior".

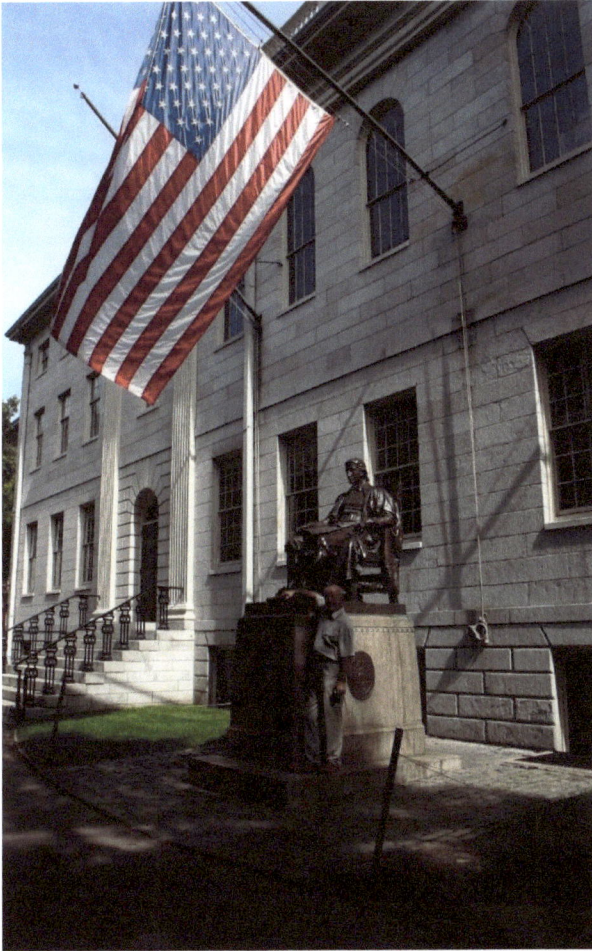

Harvard: 23 Sep 2009, on the west side of the University Hall (1813, white granite, Colonial Revival architecture, Charles Bulfinch (1763 -1844)), in the yard of Harvard University (1636, named Harvard in 1639), in Cambridge (1630, incorporated 1636, city 1846, motto: "Literis Antiquis Novis Institutis Decora." (Distinguished (Decora) for Classical (Antiquis) Learning (Literis) and New (Novis) Institutions (Institutis)), looking northeast to the statue (1884, bronze by Daniel Chester French (1850-1931)) of the founder Reverend John Harvard (1607-1638, English minister in American colonies, (his grandfather (from the mother side) Thomas Rogers (1540-1611) was an younger associate of John Shakespeare (1531-1601), father of William Shakespeare (1564-1616)), had bequeathed to the school his entire library and half of his monetary estate).

www.ingramcontent.com/pod-product-compliance
Lightning Source LLC
Chambersburg PA
CBHW041309210326

41599CB00003B/44